How to Live with a Heart Attack
(And How to Avoid One)

How to Live with

Chilton Book Company
Radnor, Pennsylvania

a Heart Attack

(And How to Avoid One)

Revised Edition

Robert A. Miller, M.D.

Library of Congress Cataloging in Publication Data
Miller, Robert Allen, 1932-
How to live with a heart attack.

1. Heart—Diseases.   2. Heart—Infarction.
I. Title.
RC672.M55   1973   616.1'2   73-11196
ISBN 0—8019—5898—9   Hardcover
ISBN 0—8019—6690—6   Paperback

34567890   654321098

Foreword

It is estimated that 20 percent of the people in the United States—40,000,000 persons—are vulnerable to heart attacks. Some 675,000 Americans will die from heart attacks this year, while twice that number will survive an attack.

The heart attack patient and his family will find an explanation in this book of the forces which lead up to his illness. They will also learn how to adjust their lives to cope successfully with their problem and, hopefully, to be active and productive.

Equally as important, the "healthy" American is given insight into the common factors which often lead to the development of heart problems during adult years. Many authorities in the field of heart disease and public health believe that a significant number of heart attacks can be prevented if people will make certain alterations in their life style at an early age. These alternate routes to longevity and health are clearly outlined in the latter portion of this book.

Hypertension and diabetes are often linked closely to coronary heart disease; these problems are explained in simple terms. Many persons confuse strokes with heart attacks which prompts the inclusion of a section dealing with the stroke problem. Important warning symptoms of serious illness are collected together in a single chapter for quick reference.

This book has not been designed to replace the guiding hand of the family physician or cardiologist; rather it is intended to supplement his task by providing detailed explanations of the various diseases and problems which patients encounter. Time does not usually permit the physician treating a heart patient to explain the situation in any detail. This book is designed to take up that explanation where the physician leaves off.

The patient who is facing heart surgery, or the person with a pacemaker, will find discussions that may clarify unanswered questions in their minds. A section also deals with systems for emergency coronary care and recent advances which have occurred through research.

This book has been written to give the reader a simplified explanation of the problems of coronary heart disease. An understanding of the situation will enable the patient to avoid hurting himself through ignorance, and will help all individuals to realize when they need medical attention.

ROBERT A. MILLER, M.D.

Contents

PULMONARY CIRCULATION

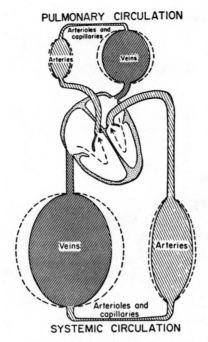

SYSTEMIC CIRCULATION

Schematic representation of the circulatory system, showing the two sides of the heart and the systemic and pulmonary circulations. From Biology, *5th ed., by Claude A. Villee, Ph.D., W. B. Saunders Co. Used by permission.*

The human heart. From Function of the Human Body, *by Arthur C. Guyton, M.D., W. B. Saunders Co. Used by permission.*

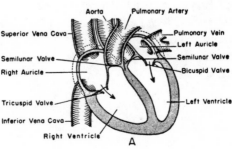

The Heart Attack

"I think it's just acute indigestion, doctor, but it won't go away." The voice came from a sixty-year-old man lying on a bed in the emergency room. "It started about four hours ago, although I had a little bit of it last night." The patient made a fist and laid it over his upper chest. "It's a bad pain right about here. At times I feel it going over to both shoulders and up into my neck."

As the doctor felt the patient's pulse, he noted that the patient's color was pale, that his skin was cool and damp, and that his breathing was slightly rapid. His story was interrupted as he paused to catch his breath.

The doctor rapidly examined the sick man and just as quickly made an electrocardiogram. His suspicion was correct. The patient had an acute myocardial infarction (a heart attack). He was wheeled away on a litter and minutes after was under the care of a special team in the Coronary Care Unit. An hour later the patient was dead. Frustration was written on the faces of the nurses and doctors who had tried to save him. If he had come in an hour or two sooner, they might have done it.

This story is a painful one that repeats itself over and over again in the hospitals of our country. "It's just indigestion, doc." Probably half of the people who have a heart attack mistake it for acute indigestion. Perhaps they think it is their heart but are afraid to admit it to themselves.

What is acute indigestion? What causes it? Strictly speaking, indigestion means incomplete or difficult digestion of food. In itself, this situation would probably not produce any symptom other than a sensation of fullness in the abdomen. People who use the term indigestion are usually referring to other things.

One common problem in the intestinal tract that is confused by people who have "heart pain" is a disorder called hiatal hernia, or a diaphragmatic hernia. This is a condition in which a small part of the stomach is able to slide up into the chest through an opening in the diaphragm. The diaphragm is the muscular structure that separates the heart and lungs from the organs of the abdomen. The esophagus, the tube that carries food from the mouth to the stomach, passes through a hole (hiatus) in the diaphragm. When a person has a diaphragmatic hernia, this normal hole is larger than it is supposed to be, and when he lies down, part of the stomach slides up into his chest. This occurs only when the person is lying down, because when he is sitting or standing, gravity pulls the stomach down low in the abdomen. If a person has symptoms from this problem, one is usually a feeling of pressure or general discomfort in the upper abdomen or the lower chest. Sometimes this hernia can produce severe pain.

The clue to the diagnosis of the hernia is that usually the pain starts sometime after the person has gone to bed after a large meal. The sooner he goes to bed after a meal, the more likely he is to experience discomfort. Furthermore, most patients find that they get relief from the pain if they sit up in bed, or better yet, if they get up and walk around. On assuming a more upright position, the stomach returns to its normal position and the pain disappears. The diagnosis of this condition is confirmed by an x-ray of the upper intestinal tract.

Another problem that may cause symptoms confused with heart pain is gallbladder disease. The gallbladder is an organ in the abdomen that lies below the liver in the right upper part of the abdomen. The gallbladder is prone to form stones and to become infected, conditions that can cause pain. Pain from diseases of the gallbladder may occur more often after meals, which gives some clue to its origin. More important in this respect is that it usually causes pain in the right upper abdomen. In fact, the upper abdomen is often tender. Vomiting is a frequent, associated symptom. Pains originating in the heart usually do not cause abdominal pain or tenderness.

Ulcers in the stomach and duodenum or gastritis (an inflammation of the stomach) might produce symptoms that some people would term indigestion. Actually, these conditions usually cause a burning pain in the uppermost part of the abdomen. The pain is usually relieved by eating, drinking milk, or taking some form of antacid. Another frequent finding in ulcer patients is that they may awaken in the middle of the night with this pain and are then able to relieve it with milk or an antacid.

An episode of food poisoning might cause indigestion for

some people. The prominent symptom here, again, is abdominal discomfort, pain, or cramps that are usually associated with or followed by vomiting or diarrhea.

These are not the symptoms that people have when they call their heart pain indigestion. Cardiac pain is usually felt in the chest and may also be felt in the shoulders, arms, neck, or jaws. Although a person with a heart attack may feel slightly nauseated and may on rare occasions vomit, these symptoms are minimal. The pain of a heart attack is located in the chest or uppermost part of the abdomen, and may gradually increase, but when it reaches its peak, it persists relentlessly. Abdominal pain from many causes is usually cyclic. The pain comes and goes; it builds up to a crescendo and then eases away.

People experience heart pain in different ways. Some persons describe the pain as having the quality of a pressure or weight upon the chest. It may feel as if someone were kneeling on the person's chest, or worse yet, as if an elephant were standing there. To other people the pain may have more of a quality of burning, piercing, or squeezing. Some people associate this pain with a pressure or feeling of distention, as if gas had built up around the heart. The pain might be temporarily relieved by belching but it always returns. Over a period of minutes or hours the pain may vary in intensity, but it has a persistent, agonizing quality.

Most people have not previously experienced such distress. This is usually a new and frightening experience. An afflicted person may feel weak and faint as he tries to stand or walk. Some will try to get relief by lying down, others by rolling around on their beds. There may or may not be a sense of suffocation accompanying the pain. If there is, the person feeling it is likely to sit up, pant for breath, loosen his collar or even walk to a window and throw it open in an attempt to get more air into his lungs.

It should be obvious to people in this predicament that something is drastically wrong. The condition is so different from indigestion and so painful that it should be clear at once that medical attention is urgently needed.

At least half of the deaths caused by a heart attack occur within the first few hours because by this time the heart has undergone an extreme injury. A damaged heart may not be able to beat properly. It may not be able to pump blood to the brain and other vital organs, and a complete state of cardiac collapse can occur within a matter of seconds or minutes. The greatest chance for survival under these circumstances is to seek immediate medical attention, preferably in a hospital. An examination by a doctor and an electrocardiogram (ECG) can frequently establish a diagnosis within a matter of minutes. If the pain is coming from an ailment in the abdomen instead of the heart, the chances are very great that medical attention would be required for pain of this severity in that location. If you are fortunate enough and no serious condition exists, at least the medical attention can relieve your pain, so you are still better off than if you had struggled through the problem by yourself at home.

Perhaps 20 percent of people who have a heart attack have minimal symptoms. Some people who have had a heart attack are never aware that something has happened. These "silent" coronaries are usually picked up in routine physical examinations by the electrocardiogram. There are certain definite signs in the ECG that are almost positive evidence of a prior heart attack. Autopsy examinations on large numbers of patients have confirmed this evidence. The probable reason for the lack of symptoms is that a blood vessel in the heart closed off gradually over a period of weeks or months rather than suddenly over a period of minutes or hours.

Another group of people may experience minor persistent symptoms that precede and herald their heart attacks. Such symptoms may include a recurring pain in the chest, neck, elbow, or even wrist or back that comes on with exertion or even at rest. The pain may have the quality of a minor toothache or pressure. The clue that something important may be happening is simple: this is usually a new experience, different from any other discomforts that the person has felt before.

Some people feel embarrassed about going to a doctor for fear that he will find nothing wrong. This is wrong in itself. It takes many years of training for a doctor to learn to make a diagnosis accurately, so certainly the average person can not be expected to be correct in the diagnosis of his own ailments even a fraction of the time. Another group of people tends to minimize all symptoms because they refuse to believe that they could possibly be sick. They have done well for so many years that it is inconceivable to them that they could suffer from a heart attack. Vanity can become a treacherous assassin. The simple truth is that 50 percent of deaths in the United States today are caused by diseases of the heart and blood vessels, and heart attacks claim 55 percent of these deaths. It can happen to you and the chances are that it eventually will.

Many hospitals in the Western world have instituted new programs in an attempt to decrease the death rate from heart attacks. Intensive care units in modern hospitals have increased the patient survival rate. In several large cities in the

United States and England, mobile coronary care units have been established to provide patients with expert attendance during their transport from home to hospital. A recent study has shown, however, that the time required to take a patient from his home to the hospital is but a fraction of the time that is wasted between the onset of the attack and actual arrival at the hospital, where positive measures can be taken to save his life. The patient usually waits hours and sometimes a day or two before he believes that something is seriously wrong and summons help. Since the greatest risk of death occurs during the first few hours of a heart attack, with the probability of death decreasing rapidly after the first day or two, it is obvious that further significant improvement in survival rates depends upon the individual himself.

2

Heart Injury and Its Consequences

The doctor said that you had a heart attack. This simple statement will be repeated over and over again in your mind in the months to follow. The important thing, however, is that you understand what this statement means. The terms that you hear will be confusing; heart attack, coronary occlusion, coronary thrombosis, and myocardial infarction are virtually synonymous. Angina pectoris is not synonymous with coronary occlusion. When a person has a heart attack, a portion of the heart muscle dies. In angina, there is a temporary insufficiency of blood flow to a part of the heart, and heart muscle death does not occur.

The heart is basically a pump that is composed primarily of muscle that expands and contracts to push blood through the body. This muscle, like all muscles in the body, must be fed with food and oxygen to function properly. If the muscle or part of the muscle is deprived of food and oxygen, serious consequences develop. Food and oxygen are carried to the heart muscle by blood flowing through the right and left coronary arteries. These are two blood vessels that arise from the aorta as soon as oxygen-rich blood has left the heart. In other words, the very first organ that the heart pumps blood to for nourishment is itself. Both coronary arteries supply a different part of the heart by way of their branches. If a main artery or one of its branches becomes obstructed for any reason, a portion of the heart muscle dies. This is a heart attack. The moment of blood vessel occlusion (blockage) and heart muscle death is usually accompanied by profound symptoms such as severe chest pain, possibly weakness, sweating, a sense of fear, and, in some instances, shortness of breath, palpitations, or fainting. If the rest of the heart can compensate during this initial phase of profound injury, the heart muscle will heal itself and the pump may again function in a near-normal fashion.

The common medical term used to describe this condition is myocardial infarction. "Myo" refers to muscle, cardial to heart, and infarction means an area of dead tissue that is caused by interruption in blood supply. This point must be emphasized—the fact that a portion of the heart muscle has died—to help you understand the immediate and long-term restrictions that this condition may impose upon you.

A great many people have the erroneous impression that a coronary thrombosis or coronary occlusion means only that an important blood vessel has been obstructed. That is correct, but it omits the consequences of heart muscle death. They have then heard that in time drugs will dissolve the blood clot that obstructs the vessel, and they then infer that they are back to "normal" again. Other people have the impression that, when a blood vessel is obstructed, "collateral blood vessels" will supply the deprived tissue with an adequate blood flow. This again is a half-truth. Collateral circulation refers to the presence of small blood vessels which communicate with the larger blood vessels. If a block occurs in a large vessel, these branches have the capacity to enlarge and shunt blood flow around the blockage to an area in need of blood. It is true that in time a blood clot may disappear, and it is also true that in time collateral blood vessels may supply with extra blood an area of the heart that lacks it. However, the diagnosis of myocardial infarction distinctly indicates that a portion of heart muscle has died before either of these two potential solutions have had time to become a reality.

In time, the area of dead muscle will be replaced by scar tissue. The time element is considered to be approximately six weeks. The reason that the patient's activity should be greatly curtailed during the six-week period is that the heart should be given a chance to form an adequate scar. The function of the heart is to pump blood throughout the body. Working muscles of the body require a greater blood flow and, therefore, impose a greater load on the heart. A person at rest requires minimal blood flow to his body muscles and, therefore, minimal heart work. A distinct possibility in the person who does not rest after a myocardial infarction is that the area of dead muscle will soften and rupture before a scar has formed. The effect is the same as punching a hole in a gas tank. When the gasoline runs out, the engine will no longer run. In the case of the human being, he dies.

Restricted activity during this critical healing phase permits the formation of a tight, effective scar. Scar tissue is incapable of performing any work. Scar tissue cannot contract to make the heart a more effective pump. A good scar, however, will draw the living muscles as close together as possible so that they can function properly without the useless part. If the heart is overworked during this period, it will tend to enlarge and a loose, thin, bulging scar will form which will hamper the work of the adjacent muscle. This loose scar is called a ventricular aneurysm.

One of the potential early complications of the myocardial infarction is heart failure. This term means that the pump is unable to move an adequate amount of blood through the body. When one portion of the heart muscle suddenly dies, the rest of the heart must take on an additional burden. This is similar to one engine of a multiengine airplane suddenly quitting in flight. If the load is not too heavy and if the remaining engines are powerful enough, the plane will continue to be airborne; otherwise the plane will crash. If the pilot has sufficient time to act, he may be able to compensate for his loss of power by throwing cargo or fuel overboard to lighten his load. The burden on the heart muscle is eased by radically reducing the activity that the entire body undertakes. This is another reason for strict rest during the early phases of a heart attack. If the heart is unable to pump an adequate blood volume, the ensuing course of events results in an engorgement of blood in the vessels of the lungs. The increased back pressure eventually results in the water portion of the blood oozing into the air spaces of the lungs, which blocks normal gas exchange. The patient literally drowns in his own fluids. The clinical picture is called pulmonary edema, which is a form of heart failure. The patient experiences this chain of events as a rapidly increasing shortness of breath.

The blood pressure of the body is maintained by a certain quantity of blood flowing through blood vessels in a given period of time. When the heart is unable to pump an adequate amount of blood, the blood pressure in the entire body will fall and a state of shock will develop. The patient experiences this as a sensation of weakness, faintness, and possibly profuse perspiration. The physician recognizes this state by a low blood pressure and a weak pulse. If this state persists for a sufficient time, the brain and other vital organs will suffer from lack of blood and irreparable damage or death may occur.

The heart normally contracts 60 to 100 times a minute, propelling blood with each contraction. The stimulus for each contraction is a discharge from nervous tissue within the heart at the same rate. The origin of these stimuli is usually the sino-atrial node, which is known as the pacemaker of the heart. However, any portion of the heart has the potential capacity for initiating a nervous impulse that can result in contraction of the heart muscle. When a portion of heart muscle dies, the remaining muscle may become very irritable and multiple areas of discharge may compete with the pacemaker, resulting in a rapid or erratic heart beat. This rhythm may be a tachycardia (rapid action) or fibrillation. If the speed of contraction is not too fast or if the rhythm of contraction is not too erratic, the heart will still pump blood effectively. If, on the other hand, the rate is too fast or the rhythm too irregular, the actual amount of blood pumped will greatly diminish and a shock-like picture will develop. The patient may experience these events as a palpitation or fluttering in his chest. The development of shock is accompanied by feelings of weakness, faintness or profuse sweating.

Physicians today are familiar with these events, and hospitals are equipped to combat many of these complicating factors. Therefore, the safest place for a person who has suffered a heart attack is in a hospital under close supervision of trained personnel. It is nostalgic to remember Grandfather's heart attack as he remained in his comfortable bed at home, visited daily by his family doctor, until it was felt safe for him to get out of bed. At that time, however, many of these serious complications were not known, and effective treatment for them was not available. Today's doctor ı ıay very well recognize over the telephone that his patient has gone into shock the third day after his heart attack, but if the patient is at home it may be too late for the doctor to do anything effective about it by the time he reaches the bedside.

The current approach to the treatment of myocardial infarction is first to get the suffering patient to the hospital quickly. After a provisional diagnosis has been made, he is moved into a special area of the hospital called a Coronary Care Unit (CCU), which is staffed and equipped expressly for this type of illness. The patient is usually under the constant supervision of doctors, nurses, and electronic machinery, all of which are focusing their attention on detecting the very first sign of any complication. If complications do develop, treatment is much more effective if it is begun early.

The development of the concept of coronary care units is of recent origin. It is the result of increasing medical knowledge and in particular of increasing knowledge about the natural history of coronary artery disease. To achieve a proper frame of reference, it is of interest that Dr. Paul White reports that in 1910 the diagnosis of a heart attack or myocardial infarct was seldom made in a general hospital in this country. His explanation is that, first, the disease itself was much less common than it is today, and, second, that doctors were not aware of the disease itself. In other words, medicine had not advanced to the point where it was commonly recognized that there was such a thing as a myocardial infarct, or what the symptoms of this illness were. By the 1920s the disease pattern was established as a distinct entity, and by World War II large numbers of patients were being treated for this condition.

By the 1960s statistics revealed that about 60 percent of the deaths of persons with atherosclerotic heart disease (the disease that causes heart attacks) were sudden deaths. Futhermore, about 70 percent of these deaths occurred during the first seven days of the illness. Just before this period, the first human being was successfully defibrillated by an electrical shock across the chest. (Ventricular fibrillation is a situation in which the heart quivers rather than beats, and it is fatal within four or five minutes.) This is a common cause of sudden death in persons with heart attacks.

Shortly after this, the technique of closed-chest cardiac massage was devised. By this is meant the application of pressure repeatedly over the chest of a person whose heart has stopped beating. With the proper application of chest compression, blood is forced into and out of the heart in a near normal fashion. The efficiency does not approach that of the normally beating heart, but enough blood can be induced to circulate to the vital organs of the body to postpone death. Formerly, if the heart stopped beating or fibrillated, death of the brain occurred in four or five minutes as mentioned above. Other forms of heart stoppage cannot be treated by defibrillation, but sometimes drugs or other forms of treatment can be used to start the heart again if the patient can be kept alive until they have a chance to take effect.

In 1767 a society for the revival of persons apparently dead by drowning was formed in Amsterdam. One of the methods recommended was mouth-to-mouth respiration. This technique was forgotten until about 1960, at which time its revival provided an improved method for giving artificial respiration.

It was now at least theoretically possible for one or preferably two persons to maintain life in a patient who had suddenly stopped breathing, or whose heart had suddenly stopped functioning. A method was now available to "buy a little time" until a person could be transported to a treatment facility, or until special forms of treatment could be brought to him.

Incidentally, no special tools are necessary to perform this cardio-pulmonary resuscitation; the only requirement is trained personnel. Both forms of assistance are usually necessary in a case of cardiac arrest or stoppage of the heart. The body must be supplied with blood that has an adequate amount of oxygen. When the heart stops functioning, breathing stops within less than a minute. Closed-chest cardiac massage is useless without artificial respiration.

To avoid any confusion, it must be pointed out that people cannot be kept alive very long with these techniques. Some hearts are too diseased to recover, and a certain percentage of cardiac arrests cannot be restarted.

Now let us look at what was happening in the hospitals in this country about ten or twelve years ago. The usual treatment for a person with a heart attack was to hospitalize him. Sometimes the patient was in a semiprivate room or ward, and sometimes he was in a private room. The more affluent frequently had private nurses. The patient's doctor would visit him once or twice a day and the nurses would check his blood pressure periodically and give him his medicines. Before the advent of cardio-pulmonary resuscitation, it was not unusual to see a patient who had sustained a heart attack suddenly become worse, and within a few minutes die. When the doctor made his morning rounds, he frequently held his breath when he checked into the nurses' station to pick up his patients' charts. He was usually thinking, "I wonder who was found dead in his bed last night."

After the advent of resuscitative measures, it then became a frustrating contest. Many doctors and nurses had been trained in the techniques of cardio-pulmonary resuscitation, but they never seemed to be at the proper patient's bedside when the poor patient needed assistance. Very little had been accomplished with these new ideas as far as decreasing patient mortality was concerned.

Since 1965 many hospitals throughout the country have established Coronary Care Units to care for patients who have had myocardial infarcts. The basic idea is to group together patients with this particular type of illness and trained personnel to handle their problems. The main ingredient of the CCU is the specially trained nurse. Some hospitals are able to have a physician in the unit at all times, but most depend upon the nurses for constant attendance. These nurses are highly motivated persons who have received extensive training in the care of cardiac patients.

The physical structure of these units is such that it is easy for the nurses on duty either to see or hear each patient. Crowding is avoided by limiting the CCU to six or eight patients. If additional beds are necessary because of the size of the hospital, then additional complete units are provided. Ideally, each patient has a private room. The doors connecting his room to the nursing area are frequently made of glass to provide optimal observation of the patient. The isolated nature of the CCU provides better control of traffic, and visitors can be held to a minimum so that the patients can get proper rest.

Electronic monitors are used to keep track of the heart beat. Electrodes (small metal plates attached to wires) are fastened to the patient's chest over the heart with adhesive. The wires usually lead to an electronic box suspended on a wall by the patient's bed, which may display the patient's electrocardiogram on an oscilloscope and also record his heart rate. Another machine on the wall may be connected to a blood pressure cuff on the patient's arm. This automatically records the blood pressure at intervals of time, and sends the information to the nurses' station, which is usually situated centrally to the patient rooms.

The data from each patient are recorded or displayed in a variety of ways. There may be one or more central oscilloscopes to display the electrocardiogram and one or more banks of instruments that keep track of the heartbeat and blood pressure. Additional instruments are sometimes used that regularly record the patients' temperature, respiration, and so on. These mechanical devices have alarms built into them that will signal the nurses on duty if the patient's blood pressure falls, or if the pulse slows or speeds up too much. The nurses are trained to interpret the electrocardiograms that reveal whether or not the patient's heart is beating normally, even if the pulse is the correct speed.

The design of the unit keeps the nurses in close contact with the patients. This fact, coupled with the electronic sensing devices, ensures that if a heart stoppage or fibrillation occurs it is immediately detected. A doctor is summoned, but the nurses begin whatever resuscitative measures are necessary. Equipment is at hand to defibrillate the patient if this is required. The nurses have been trained to perform this function if necessary. Mouth-to-mouth breathing can be performed, but special machines are also at hand to provide artificial respiration.

The result of these programs is that the mortality rate in myocardial infarction has been reduced by 30 to 50 percent of what it formerly was.

3
Atherosclerosis—
The Cause of Heart Attacks

The basic cause for approximately 90 percent of myocardial infarctions is arteriosclerosis, or "hardening of the arteries." This word, arteriosclerosis, is the family name describing several disease processes. You may, at times, run across the term atherosclerosis, which is the specific member of the family that is affecting your blood vessels. For our purposes, however, we can consider that arteriosclerosis and atherosclerosis are synonymous.

This disease can affect blood vessels in several ways, but the common result is the narrowing of the arteries and therefore a decrease in the amount of blood that can flow through the arteries in a given time. Arteries in many different parts of the body may be affected by atherosclerosis. If the primary area involved is in the coronary arteries (the two arteries that feed the heart), a myocardial infarction or angina pectoris may develop, the former, if actual death of heart muscle has occurred. If the process involves primarily the blood vessels supplying the brain, a stroke may be the outcome. The same disease may affect the blood vessels of the legs and result in symptoms ranging from pain in the muscles of the calf on walking to gangrene of the toes or a greater portion of the foot or leg.

An easy way to visualize the effect of this disease of blood vessels is to think of the problem that results inside water pipes that have carried hard water for many years. The inside of the pipe becomes coated with a limey substance, and the opening or bore of the pipe becomes progressively narrower. Obviously the amount of water that flows through the pipe is progressively diminished. Atherosclerosis does not cause such a uniform narrowing of the blood vessel. The process occurs in distinct patches. It may be easier to visualize this if one were to think of a garden hose that had lima beans glued to the inside of the hose at intervals. The diameter of the hose would be narrowed at each spot where a lima bean was found, but in between the beans the diameter would be normal. Such intermittent narrowing of the blood vessel does not necessarily decrease the effective blood flow because the blood flow may merely speed up as it passes each obstruction.

A person could therefore have a considerable amount of atherosclerosis in his blood vessels without producing any symptoms. As a matter of fact, persons in their fifties and sixties who are examined after death frequently are found to have significant amounts of atherosclerosis in their heart or in the blood vessels that lead to their brain or to their limbs, but they may never have had any symptoms that suggested disease in these areas. You might say that Lady Luck had a great deal to do with the determination of who would or who would not have angina pectoris or a heart attack. If the atherosclerosis in your blood vessels is not of a critical degree or if the patches do not occur in critical areas, you may get away with a great deal of blood vessel damage without ever being aware of it.

In this general area of disease, several things may happen to produce the startling event that we know as a heart attack. In about 50 percent of cases of myocardial infarction, a thrombosis has occurred which completely blocked a blood vessel. A thrombosis is a medical term for a blood clot. The blood clot frequently forms on or near one of these patches of atherosclerosis. In some cases, a patch of atherosclerosis becomes detached from the wall of the artery and is carried further down the blood vessel until it completely occludes the artery. In some instances, for unknown reasons, a small hemorrhage develops beneath the plaque and pushes it out to obstruct the lumen (passageway) of the artery. The end effect in all these instances is obstruction of the artery with an obvious deficit of blood flow to the muscle that lies beyond the area of obstruction.

Some hearts that have been examined after a fatal heart attack reveal no actual obstruction of the blood vessel, only a narrowing of the artery. In this circumstance, how did the infarction develop? It is difficult, if not impossible, to know exactly what happened, but this may be what occurs. Most of us are familiar with the function of gasoline engines. Many of us have at one time or another tinkered with our engines and are aware that if the gas line between the fuel tank and the fuel pump were kinked difficulty would arise. The engine might run satisfactorily at idling speed, or even when the automobile was running at 20 or 30 miles per hour. But at some critical point, say 40 miles per hour, enough gas would not pass through the obstruction and the engine would falter.

In the automobile there is no great problem because if

the engine falters the car merely slows down. In the human mechanism, however, a different result may occur. If a person were doing heavy work, the muscles in his arms and legs would be burning up oxygen and food at a rapid rate. These substances are supplied by the blood stream, and the normal course of events is for the heart to pump a greater amount of blood into the blood vessels to supply the working muscles. When the heart pumps a greater quantity of blood, it, too, is working harder and requires a greater amount of oxygen and food. These energy substances must be delivered through the coronary arteries. If the coronary arteries are narrowed and are unable to deliver adequate amounts of food and oxygen to the heart muscle during total body exercise, and if the total body work and the demands upon the heart continue despite inadequate nourishment of the heart muscle, that portion of the heart muscle supplied by a narrowed coronary artery could, figuratively speaking, burn itself out.

We believe that when the heart receives inadequate food and oxygen, it sends a signal to our conscious mind in the form of chest pain. If the period of deficient blood flow is of short duration, no damage will occur to the heart muscle. If this deficiency is prolonged beyond a critical period, the heart tissue will die. This, again, is essentially the difference between angina pectoris and a myocardial infarction. Angina pectoris is known to the patient as a chest pain that is usually of just several minutes duration. Although it may occur when a person is at rest, it usually happens when a person is active or after he has eaten a heavy meal. The person who has the pain usually stops what he is doing, or lies down, or takes a nitroglycerine tablet and within a few minutes the pain is relieved. When the person stopped walking, he decreased the demands that his leg muscles were placing on his heart and the heart could rest temporarily. This is probably why the pain stopped. When a person takes a nitroglycerine tablet, the drug temporarily increases the nourishment of the heart and, again, the pain stops. If the pain persists for many minutes or hours despite rest or nitroglycerine, it is likely that a complete occlusion has occurred and actual muscle death and myocardial infarction are in process.

We have just discussed the mechanism of a coronary occlusion or a heart attack and mentioned that atherosclerosis was the basic culprit. Let us examine this process in more detail.

The patches of atherosclerosis which protrude into the interior of arteries are accumulations of fats, cholesterol, and calcium, and scar tissue induced by such foreign substances. These patches, or plaques, are not entirely on the surface of the vessel but usually extend deep into the wall of the artery, so much so that if one were removed, the vessel wall would be thinner and weaker in that location.

Arterial plaques apparently begin to develop at an early age. During the Korean War, autopsies performed on United States soldiers who died of combat wounds revealed that 20 percent of these men in their early twenties already had significant amounts of atherosclerosis in their coronary arteries. Plaques have even been found in the coronary arteries of children under ten years of age. Women tend to develop these lesions at a later age than men, being protected by some unknown factor (female hormone—estrogen?) until after their menopause, at which time they accelerate the development of atherosclerotic plaques and almost catch up to men in the frequency of heart attacks. Heart attacks do occur in men in their twenties and early thirties, but are much more common in the forty to fifty age group.

Certain things appear to accelerate the development of

atherosclerosis. Cigarette smokers have a definite increased risk. People who are overweight and sedentary have a greater risk. High blood pressure and diabetes are both factors that increase the risk and the likelihood of developing the disease at a younger age.

The word cholesterol is beginning to produce the same effect on some people as the mention of "Internal Revenue." The two terms are probably equally maligned and misunderstood by the public. Cholesterol is a type of fat found in certain foods and also produced in the human body. Cholesterol has many important functions in the body, the most important being to supply the basic structure upon which body hormones are produced. Hormones are internal secretions which are essential for bodily function. Sex distinction is one hormonal effect.

In some diseases, such as hypothyroidism (inadequate production of thyroid hormone), an excess of cholesterol is produced by the body and there is also found an accelerated development of atherosclerosis. Certain scientific studies, particularly in Sweden, have demonstrated that an increased cholesterol content of the diet is associated with a higher death rate from myocardial infarction or heart attacks. From these facts and other information a hypothesis has developed that maybe cholesterol is an important culprit in the cause of atherosclerosis. Large-scale studies are underway in the United States at this time to attempt to define the relationship between diet, cholesterol, heart attacks, and death from blood vessel diseases, and to arrive at methods to achieve dietary and drug control of blood cholesterol levels.

Many questions remain to be answered. Several tentative conclusions can be drawn that time may substantiate. First, since the disease process appears to start very early in life, it makes sense to consider altering the diets (and thereby the cholesterol in the blood) of children and young adults. In oldsters, the disease is usually far advanced and thus more difficult to reverse. Second, certain people are not able to handle cholesterol and fats as well as are others, but blood tests are now available which can identify these high-risk persons, and they may be helped by more vigorous dietary plans or by certain drugs. Third, many other factors besides cholesterol and diet are involved in the development of atherosclerosis, and undue emphasis should not be placed on these two.

If a person has high blood cholesterol and other body fats, a low cholesterol diet may help to correct this condition. The usual diet precludes egg yolks, butter, milk, cream, cheese, ice cream, meat fat, and shellfish. Some people, however, appear to produce undesirable fats (such as triglycerides) within their own bodies from simple sugars, such as those found in sugar, fruit, and alcoholic drinks. In general, obesity is associated with higher cholesterol levels, and one universal way to reduce blood cholesterol is to reduce body weight. A physician can best help the patient to determine whether he needs a strict cholesterol diet, weight reduction, or a decrease in sugar and alcohol.

A more extensive review of cholesterol and other risk factors involved in developing heart attacks is contained in the chapter entitled "Can I Prevent a Heart Attack?" The same factors apply in preventing a second heart attack as apply in preventing the first.

4

Healing the Wound

The burning question in minds of men and women during and immediately after a heart attack is, "Will I be able to go back to work?" "Will I be able to take care of my family?" It is difficult, if not impossible, for your doctor to tell you exactly what you will be able to do when you eventually leave the hospital, but if you understand the problem involved you may be able to help yourself.

We must go back to the basic fact that your heart is a pump designed to pump blood. This muscular structure in a young adult has a phenomenal reserve capacity. On demand it may be able to pump seven or eight times as much blood per minute as it does when you are asleep. In other words, during extreme exercise your heart may be able to deliver 30 quarts of blood per minute to your body compared to the four quarts per minute that may be pumped during complete rest. As the years pass, the body ages and we are all aware that we no longer have, for example, the muscular strength that we had when we were twenty years old, nor at age sixty do we have the sense of sight or smell that we had when we were twenty years old.

In a similar way the reserve capacity of your heart may be diminished by the process of aging. A person at age fifty may have a reserve capacity of five times, or possibly six times, the resting level of blood flow. We have stated previously that the result of a coronary thrombosis or myocardial infarction is the death of heart muscle. There is less heart muscle to pump the blood after a myocardial infarction than there was before the incident. The reserve capacity of the heart must, therefore, be diminished. This is the determining factor that will decide what you will or will not be able to do after your heart attack. If enough functioning muscle remains, you may be able to do practically the same things that you were able to do before your heart attack. This, of course, is particularly true if you had a large reserve capacity.

The primary symptoms that you may recognize if you exceed your reserve capacity will probably be chest pain in the form of angina pectoris, fatigue, or shortness of breath on exertion. It is essential that the person who has recovered from a heart attack understand the factors that increase the demands upon the heart if he is to avoid difficulty and make the most of his physical impairment. The main factors that result in increased heart work are exercise, eating, emotional excitement, and extremes of temperature. Let us examine each of these in detail.

When you exercise, as for example, taking a walk or hammering a nail, the muscles of your legs and arms are active and are doing work. This work demands increased food and oxygen to nourish the muscles of your legs and arms. Food and oxygen are carried to the muscles by blood that is pumped by your heart. Exercise, therefore, increases the work of the heart.

The process of eating, and in particular digesting food, requires increased blood flow to the stomach and intestines. When food enters your stomach, the muscles of the stomach contract to mix the food with digestive juices and to propel the food to the intestinal tract. The intestinal tract also contracts to mix the food and to propel it further along. Great quantities of stomach acid and various digestive juices are poured into the intestinal tract to aid in digestion of the consumed food. These juices are produced by glands all of which depend upon blood for their raw materials. The production of digestive juices and the action of the intestinal muscles, therefore, require increased blood flow which must be supplied by the heart.

A state of excitement or tension, anger, rage, or fear also results in increased heart work because these situations stimulate the adrenal glands, which produce adrenaline. The adrenaline circulates throughout the body and prepares the body for an emergency such as a fight or a flight (running away). The action of adrenaline upon the heart is to increase the rate of heart contraction and the work of the heart. A person who is frightened or angry, therefore, may have a heart that is working just as hard as if the man were actually running at full speed down the street.

Most of us know that the body temperature is maintained near 98.6 degrees Fahrenheit. This temperature is held rather constantly by the body because all systems are geared to function best at this temperature level. When we are exposed to heat or cold, our body attempts to adjust itself to these circumstances and to maintain an internal temperature as near to normal as possible. We are familiar with the process of shivering when we are chilled. Shivering results from a rapid contraction of muscles in various parts of the body. This muscular contraction produces heat which warms the blood and helps maintain a constant body temperature. When we are hot, on the other hand, the body compensates by perspiring and radiating heat from the skin surface. The blood flow to the skin increases, carrying body heat to the surface blood vessels from which it can be radiated. The process of perspiration requires the production of water, which surfaces to the skin, and by the process of evaporation allows the body to lose heat. This slightly salty water is produced by sweat glands through the basic operation of increased blood flow to these organs. Therefore, a person who is exposed to a hot or a cold environment has increased heart work.

Your heart may be strong enough to perform any of these functions singly, but if it is called upon to perform several simultaneously, it may not be able to do so and trouble will result.

The worst possible combination would be for a cardiac patient to eat a large meal at noon, go outside immediately and dig in his garden in the hot sun, and then become enraged with his wife or neighbor over some trifle. To understand the reasons for this also helps explain the common news items in our papers about persons who developed a heart attack while shoveling snow. With these facts in mind, the post-coronary patient can save himself a great deal of trouble. To be forewarned is to be forearmed. A basic underlying rule for such patients should be to avoid unnecessary mental or physical strains.

We cannot do a great deal to change the basic situation. It is impossible for us to replace the scarred tissue remnant of previously living muscle with new muscle. The changes that have occurred as a result of the aging process cannot be reversed. Although in some instances the coronary blood vessels can be operated upon and blood flow can be increased through the vessels, in many instances this cannot be done. How fortunate it is, indeed, that the patient may have a powerful weapon at his disposal to overcome his own situation and increase his life span. That weapon is moderation.

My grandfather was a farmer who used a Model T truck to transport his produce to market for 35 years. I marveled at the tenacity of this ancient vehicle and the faithfulness with which it pulled its load of potatoes and strawberries over the small hills of West Virginia. The truck was so old that its license plate was painted on the hood. It was considered an antique and did not require plates. "How can this truck still serve you after all these years?", I once asked the old man. The answer was a statement of basic mechanical fact. "Each year I make the load a little lighter and if I pamper the truck this way it will still do its job."

The person who weighs 200 pounds demands more from his heart when he walks down the street at a leisurely pace than the person who weighs 150 pounds. Each of those 50 additional pounds requires increased blood flow. A great many coronary patients in our society are grossly overweight. If this excess weight is lost, if the person is trimmed down to bare muscle and bone, he can increase his reserve heart capacity and thereby be able to do a great deal more without symptoms of cardiac trouble. When your doctor tells you to lose 20 or 30 pounds, he means it for your good. The rewards are enormous and may possibly be measured in months and years of additional life.

Carefully planned exercise is another tool that can be used to improve the heart after a myocardial infarct. After the healing process is complete, a graded exercise program prescribed by the patient's physician will frequently increase a person's cardiac reserve. This has been demonstrated by measuring the pulse rate of a person at the beginning of an exercise program and some weeks later finding a slower pulse with the same or greater amounts of exercise. The heart, like other muscles in the body, responds to regular exercise by a strengthening of its fibers and by an increase in its efficiency. It is also possible that regular exercise can stimulate small blood vessels in the heart to become larger.

Some people are fortunate in having very small areas of muscle death as a result of a myocardial infarct. These individuals heal their hearts more rapidly and may have practically no decrease in their original cardiac reserve. They may be able to return rather quickly to their former work without any significant evidence that they were ill. This is a story with a happy ending. But even these people should have a good evaluation of their total physical and emotional situation in order to discover any factors that may be modified to attempt to prevent future myocardial infarcts. One infarct provides evidence that atherosclerosis exists in the coronary arteries. Although there may have been only one diseased area in the arteries, there probably are more potential areas of trouble, and additional myocardial infarcts will result in the death of more heart tissue.

Doctors try very hard to avoid making their patients "cardiac cripples." These are people who have survived a heart attack but who are terrified of a subsequent attack. In extreme cases they withdraw from their work and any form of physical or emotional stress. They are literally waiting around to die and fearing that they will.

In summary, then, if you have recovered from a heart attack, use a rational approach to your situation. In the vast majority of cases there is something constructive that you can do to improve your general health and to prevent further heart trouble. If your doctor advises that you quit smoking, lose weight, stick to a low cholesterol diet, take medicine for high blood pressure, and exercise regularly—do it. You may very well end up being a stronger, healthier, and happier individual than you were before your heart attack. Don't sit around and wait for the world to end.

5
Surgery and Coronary Artery Disease

Surgeons throughout the world have devised a number of approaches to diseases of the coronary arteries. Fortunately, surgery is not necessary for most people who have these diseases.

Persons who have recently sustained a heart attack or who have developed angina pectoris should be carefully evaluated for the presence of any factors that could have predisposed them to the event. One or more causative factors are frequently found that can be altered to reduce the patient's chances of developing additional trouble. The surgical attack to this problem is usually aimed at removing obstructions or bypassing obstructions in the coronary arteries. The goal is to improve the blood supply to the heart. The angina patient has a narrowing in his coronary arteries at one or more places, with inadequate blood flow beyond the obstruction. The heart attack patient has a blood vessel blockage that produced heart damage, and he hopes to avoid additional blood vessel occlusion and a subsequent heart attack.

When considering medical versus surgical therapy for coronary artery disease, two important points must be kept in mind. First, a localized artery narrowing of 80 percent may still allow an almost normal quantity of blood to pass by through the compensatory mechanism of increased flow. This phenomenon occurs in nature when a wide, lazy river narrows down to a gorge and the water rushes through the narrows. Second, during the process of removing or bypassing obstructions in the coronary arteries by surgery, only parts of the total arterial system are repaired. It is impossible to widen all the narrowed areas.

I have frequently seen men or women recently afflicted with angina pectoris who have obtained complete relief from pain during certain activities by giving up cigarette smoking. These activities were previously incapacitating, since they predictably caused severe chest pressure. The exact reason for this is not known, but nicotine probably causes blood vessels throughout the body to constrict, or narrow down. The heart then must work harder to pump blood through these tinier channels at a higher pressure. Removing the nicotine results in a relaxation and widening of the blood vessels and decreased heart work.

A large number of patients are also found to have high blood pressure associated with their angina or heart attack. Hypertension probably preceded the onset of heart disease and may have accelerated the development of coronary artery narrowing. Effective drugs are available that will lower most blood pressures, and it is very common to find that a person has less angina after his pressure returns to near normal. Similarly, a person who has hypertension and develops a myocardial infarct is less likely to have a subsequent infarct if elevated blood pressure is brought under control.

Obesity is a common finding among heart attack victims. The heart's work is increased with every pound of extra weight that a person carries above his bare minimum weight. A person who is 30 pounds overweight may decrease the amount of work that his heart performs by 20 percent if he reduces his weight to ideal levels. This reduction of heart work may very well compensate for the amount of heart muscle that has been lost by a heart attack. An obese heart attack patient may therefore end up no worse off after a heart attack if he can shrink his size. The angina patient has chest pain because, at a certain level of body activity, his coronary arteries cannot supply enough blood to the heart muscle. The heart muscle will need less blood to function if he loses weight because the heart will not have to pump as much blood to his thinner body during the same amount of exercise.

A smaller group of people has difficulty with angina because of periodic episodes of rapid heart beat. In these individuals the normal heart beat may be temporarily replaced by an abnormal rhythm that races the heart. These heart rhythms are called tachycardias. The tachycardias are distinguished from one another by different appearances on the electrocardiogram and, for example, may be variously called supraventricular tachycardia, atrial tachycardia, nodal tachycardia, ventricular tachycardia, atrial fibrillation, or atrial flutter.

The reason that these tachycardias may cause angina or chest discomfort is centered on the fact that the heart must fill itself with blood after every contraction that has emptied it of blood. As the heart rate speeds up, the time available for filling decreases. Eventually, at a certain speed, heart filling falls below normal. and therefore the heart is not pumping as much blood out to the circulation as it should. The coronary arteries are not filled properly and the heart is being deprived of adequate nourishment. Chest discomfort follows. A variety of drugs such as digitalis, pronestyl, quinidine, and propanolol can be prescribed to help control and prevent these abnormal heart rhythms. Therefore, if the patient were having angina pains as a consequence of a too rapid heartbeat, he may have significantly less angina with the control of this phenomenon.

For people who do not fall into these categories, drugs are available that may still favorably influence their angina and the course of their disease. These drugs either increase the circulation of blood to the heart muscle directly by enlarging the smaller blood vessels of the heart or decrease heart work by influencing factors outside the heart.

We have seen that many persons who develop angina pectoris or who have heart attacks have causative factors present that can be modified to alleviate their discomfort and probably prolong their lives. The surgical approach to the problem is applied to patients who are not improved by the measures mentioned. The next step in evaluating these patients for surgical help is to define as exactly as possible the areas of narrowing inside their coronary arteries. This is accomplished by taking pictures of the inside of these arteries. The procedure is termed coronary arteriography. This examination is relatively safe when it is performed by physicians who are experienced in the technique. A small hollow tube is inserted into an artery in one arm or the groin. The tube can be seen in a fluoroscope as it is advanced through the arteries to the heart. The tip of the tube is guided into the beginning of each coronary artery in the aorta just above the heart itself. A dye is injected into the tubing and flows into the coronary artery. At the same time x-ray pictures are taken very rapidly, usually with a motion picture camera. The end result is a series of pictures of the heart that show it beating, and that show the progression of blood through the coronary arteries that lie around the heart. Partial obstructions or blockages of the arteries are usually easily seen.

The surgeon and cardiologists then study these films and decide whether or not an operation can help that particular patient. If the arteries are narrowed at only one or two places, it may be possible to repair that one segment of vessel. If the arteries have multiple occlusions and generalized narrowing, it may be impossible to bypass or to clean out the interior of the vessels.

Ronald S. is a 39-year-old farmer who developed angina six months before he was considered for coronary artery surgery. He was not overweight, nor did he have high blood pressure. After his doctor had established diagnosis by means of a complete physical examination and various tests, he recommended that Ronald stop smoking cigarettes. His father had died at age 45 of acute indigestion, and an older brother, who was also a farmer, had died after his second heart attack at age 42. Ronald raised hogs and for years had enjoyed a diet rich in pork, as well as in butter and ice cream. His cholesterol level was 450 mg%, compared with a normal range of 150 to 250 mg%. (Cholesterol is measured as the quantity in milligrams found in each 100 cubic centimeters of blood plasma.) His doctor felt that his dietary habits, 30 cigarettes per day, and a strong family history of heart disease had produced his coronary atherosclerosis. Despite the abstinence from tobacco and a good program of medicines to improve his heart function, Ronald's angina grew progressively worse and he was unable to work his farm. The future appeared dismal for him and his family.

Coronary arteriograms were performed and he was found to have a 90 percent narrowing of the right coronary artery within one inch of its origin from the aorta and a second narrowing of 80 percent two inches further along the line. The patient accepted the risks of surgery and was in the operating room the following week. After his chest was opened, an artificial heart-lung machine was attached and his own heart was stopped by an injection of a drug. The heart-lung machine was now supplying his body with blood and his heart was lying quietly, ready for repair. A decision had been made to attack the high obstruction with a patch graft. The artery was opened and the plaque of white atherosclerosis was teased out. If the artery had been sutured closed at this point, the stitches would have pulled it together too tightly and another narrowing would have resulted. Instead, a piece of vein was removed from his leg and a small, elliptical patch was sewed to the edges of his coronary artery where the original incision had been made to remove the atherosclerotic plaque. The result was that the repaired artery now ballooned slightly where the patch had been sewn. The inside diameter of the artery was now greater than it had ever been.

The second area of obstruction was longer and the vessel was smaller at this point, so the team had elected to do an endarterectomy here (that is, to open the artery and remove the inner lining). Another incision was made just above the second area of narrowing. A small, thin, pointed instrument was introduced into the vessel to separate the patch of obstructing material from the vessel wall. The instrument was advanced down the artery as far as possible and then a plug of material two inches long was drawn out through the small incision. Another technique for accomplishing this maneuver is to use a jet of carbon dioxide directed through a needle to dissect the atheromatous material from the vessel wall. The incision was carefully closed without a patch. The patient's heart was restarted by the injection of another drug into the heart, and he was disconnected from the heart-lung machine. The chest was closed and the operation terminated.

Ronald had no postoperative complications and no further chest pain. Two months after surgery he was able to return to work on his farm. He realized that trouble could develop all over again, however, and did not resume smoking. His doctor was able to help him rearrange his eating habits, and his cholesterol fell to normal levels.

One of the earliest operations to improve blood flow to the heart was the Vineberg procedure. In this operation, an artery that does not normally feed the heart is implanted into the heart muscle. The donor artery is usually one of the two internal mammary arteries that lie inside the chest cage running downward from the neck toward the abdomen; alternatively, an intercostal artery is used. The intercostal arteries lie between the ribs originating in the back from the aorta. The body does not miss these arteries if they are redirected to the heart. Other adjacent arteries take over their functions. The internal mammary artery is not disturbed at its origin. The terminal six or eight inch length is dissected from the chest wall. The end of the artery is tied closed, but the short side branches that were cut to free the main artery are left open. An instrument is used to force a tunnel through the muscular wall of the heart in an area of the heart that has been shown by the arteriograms to need additional blood flow. The tunnel runs parallel to the surface of the heart. The end of the internal mammary artery is pulled through the tunnel and the tunnel is closed over the artery. The heart now has an additional blood vessel to feed it blood (or two if both internal mammary arteries were used). The blood flows through the side branches of the internal mammary artery directly into the heart muscle, and the pressure gradually forces the blood between the tiny muscle fibers and eventually back into the interior chambers of the heart, where it rejoins the rest of the circulating blood. Coronary arteriograms that have been performed several years after an internal mammary implant have shown that in some persons the new artery eventually joins up with branches of the patient's own coronary arteries.

The Vineberg operation never reached great popularity because in the majority of cases, the results were much less than desired.

The favorite operation at the present time is the saphenous vein coronary bypass procedure. In this surgery, a vein from the leg is removed and a piece of this is attached to the aorta near the origin of the coronary artery. A hole is made in the aorta and the vein end is sewed around the hole. The other end of the vein is attached to the coronary artery beyond the area of narrowing. A passageway joins the two vessels. The vein is now able to shunt blood directly from the aorta to the coronary artery beyond the obstructing plaque of atherosclerosis.

Dr. W. Dudley Johnson, associate professor of surgery at the Medical College of Wisconsin, has reported that 90 percent of his patients with angina pectoris have had relief of their chest pain for up to three and a half years after surgery.

In those patients who have not had their hearts weakened by one or more heart attacks, the mortality from surgery is low—on the order of from two to three percent.

The operation's popularity is attested to by the fact that over 20,000 such operations have been performed in the United States in the past twelve months. The *Medical World News* (13:39–50, 1972) predicts that, "on the basis of current popularity, vein grafting will become the most frequently performed operation in America. . . . " The operation is technically appealing to surgeons because several obstructions may be bypassed during a single surgery. Many patients receive two grafts, and as many as six bypasses have been used in a single person.

Despite the enthusiasm of some of its proponents, many cardiologists are advising caution with the operation. Although the mortality in some studies is only two or three percent, other people have reported mortalities as high as 20 percent. This statistic, of course, varies with the severity of the individual's illness at the time of surgery. The best candidates for any surgery have not had prior heart attacks. A person whose heart is scarred from multiple attacks usually has a poorly functioning heart muscle, and increasing the blood flow in specific areas of these hearts will not improve the basic situation. Scarred heart tissue cannot be made to perform any better by increasing the flow of blood to it. This type of patient also has a very high risk factor with bypass surgery.

A second problem is that, one year after surgery, 20 percent of the vein grafts have become occluded—no blood flows through them. This is the main reason that some authorities advise caution. Since the operation has not been around long enough to determine the long term results, no one knows how many of the grafts will still be functioning after five or ten years.

It does appear, however, that in properly selected patients, the quality of life may be improved—they will no longer have disabling angina pectoris. The question that remains unanswered is, what effect will the surgery have on the quantity of life—will life be prolonged? Long-term results require long-term evaluation, and these studies are in process.

Drs. H. Edward Garrett, Edward W. Dennis, and Michael E. DeBakey from the Baylor College of Medicine in Houston recently reported a case in the February 1973 *Journal of the American Medical Association* that is pertinent to our discussion. The subject was a patient who had had in 1964 what was possibly the first successful vein bypass graft. The patient was then 42 years old. In 1971, he was restudied, coronary arteriograms were taken, and the tests verified that his graft was still open and functioning. The examination also revealed that he had sustained a heart attack after the operation and that the other coronary arteries had become progressively narrowed during the passage of time. Thus, a bypass operation is not a guarantee that the patient will have no further heart attacks. Actually, heart attacks occur in from 10 to 20 percent of all patients having the operation.

This study also points out another fact that must be emphasized: the operation does not protect the patient from continuing problems with the further narrowing of coronary arteries caused by atherosclerosis. The patient does not gain a "protective shield" against atherosclerosis, and he must still control certain factors (hypertension, diet, and cigarette smoking) if he is to reduce the chance of further damage to his arteries.

The main use for this operation today is in cases of angina pectoris which cannot be controlled by medical means and in which the patient does not have a badly scarred heart. Medical control includes those methods that have been discussed earlier in this chapter.

Dr. Bernard Lown of the Peter Bent Brigham Hospital in Boston believes that medical treatment can improve the vast majority of patients with angina pectoris. Of the patients that he sees in referral, only about one percent fall into the category of surgical candidates.

Some physicians have attempted this operation on patients who were considered, because of greatly increased frequency and intensity of their angina, to be on the verge of a heart attack, and the procedure has been tried within a few hours of the patient actually sustaining a heart attack. The results are difficult to evaluate at this time; additional studies will be necessary.

In evaluating the results of this operation, the outcome of patients who do not have surgery must be considered. Some studies have shown that only three percent of all patients with angina die each year, and surgical statistics will have to better this before all cardiologists agree that surgery is the answer to the coronary problem.

Cardiac surgeons have at their disposal other methods to help some patients who have already suffered heart attacks. We discussed in an earlier chapter the healing of the heart after a myocardial infarct. We said that a scar is formed in the area of the heart muscle where the infarct and the resulting death of heart muscle have occurred. In some persons, a very weak and flabby scar forms, which will eventually develop into a balloon so that, with each heartbeat, the scar billows outward like a sail. This ballooning effect greatly decreases the efficiency of the heart as a pump. With the assistance of a heart-lung machine, surgeons can remove this flabby scar (called an aneurysm) and sew the heart muscle back together again. Another scar forms at the site of the incision, but this time the scar is narrow and tight, thanks to the sutures.

A heart attack can result in internal perforations of the heart, called septal defects. These have been successfully repaired using patches of synthetic material. A heart valve may also be damaged in certain cases of myocardial infarction. When this occurs, the valve can be sewn back into its normal shape and form or can be replaced by an artificial valve.

Finally, a group of surgeons in Canada has experimented with operative removal of the dead heart muscle within hours or days of the onset of the myocardial infarct. This maneuver was designed to attempt to save those desperately ill patients who had such massive areas of heart destruction that they were dying of heart failure. This procedure is still being evaluated in regard to risk versus benefits. It is mentioned to give the reader an idea of the diverse avenues that surgery is devising to cope with the problem.

It is fortunate that surgery is not the standard form of treatment for all patients with angina pectoris or myocardial infarcts. The magnitude of the problem would overwhelm the surgical facilities of this country. The situation would be similar to that which we would see in the automotive repair business if every person in the United States were allowed to purchase only one automobile in his lifetime and had to have this one car repaired time after time.

The only practical solution to the problem is to devise some accurate and simple test that will identify persons with significant coronary atherosclerosis and then treat these people with a drug that will reverse the atheromatous process. This drug has not yet been discovered or identified, but experimental work is proceeding along these lines. A basic component of human and animal connective tissue and cartilage is called chondroitin-sulfuric acid. Initial experiments with this substance suggests that this may be the drug we are seeking, but extensive experiments over a period of several years will be necessary to prove or disprove its usefulness.

6

Pacemakers

The four women had finished lunch and were about to start their bridge session. Susan remarked that they all must have enjoyed the lunch because there wasn't a scrap left on their plates. The words had just been spoken when Helen, who was sitting opposite, saw Susan's face go blank, and then Susan slumped to the floor, her forehead missing the edge of the table by inches. The women jumped out of their chairs dumbfounded and saw Susan lying on the floor unconscious. Before they could do anything, Susan started to recover, sat up, and said that she had bruised her knee. She said that she felt all right, then sat in her chair and insisted that they continue with the cards.

The next day Susan saw her doctor and related the story to him. She was more concerned now, realizing that something strange had happened. Five years previously she had been hospitalized with a mild heart attack that had partially damaged the conduction system of her heart, producing a left bundle branch block (similar to a damaged nerve). Her doctor had been watching her for any change that might indicate that she was developing further trouble. The fainting spell was the clue. After he had taken an electrocardiogram, the doctor told Susan that she had fainted because her heart had momentarily stopped beating, and that the faint was due to a lack of blood flowing to her brain. Fortunately, her heart started to beat again on its own within seconds, and she had not suffered permanent damage. If her heart had paused for three or four minutes, however, she might have suffered permanent brain damage, or even have died. The doctor recommended that she have an artificial pacemaker installed in her heart.

The heart has its own natural "pacemaker"—a system inside the heart that functions in much the same way as an electrical circuit in a house or automobile. Impulses develop periodically and are carried throughout the heart by "wires" (nerves) which end in the small heart muscle fibers. These impulses signal the muscle to contract. The origin of the normal impulse is the sino-atrial or S-A node in the right atrium. This pacemaking structure can be likened to the distributor in an auto engine, which sends signals to the spark plugs and causes them to fire.

There are only two main "wires" in the heart which link the natural pacemaker to the ventricles, which pump the blood. Just as in a two-cylinder engine, if one of the spark plug wires were cut, only a single spark plug would fire. If both spark plug wires were cut, even though the distributor still functioned, the engine would be dead.

The two wires (nerves) in the heart are called the right and left bundle branches. When one of the wires is not functioning, the problem is identified by the term right or left bundle branch block. A typical electrocardiographic picture is produced by these malfunctions which, of course, aids in the diagnosis. If both of the wires are nonfunctional, the patient is said to have a complete heart block. In this circumstance the natural pacemaker will still be functioning, but the message will not be transmitted to the ventricles. The ventricles will either not beat at all, or a secondary natural pacemaker in the ventricle itself may take over and initiate a periodic heart beat. This standby secondary pacemaker is always very slow, producing only 30 to 40 beats per minute, which may or may not be adequate to provide blood flow in sufficient quantity to allow the body to function. In some instances, the primary natural pacemaker fails—and no impulse is then generated to flow through the wires, a circumstance called sinus arrest.

Interruptions in function may occur suddenly and be permanent, or may occur intermittently, with normal heart function in the interim. The usual symptom is faintness or fainting due to inadequate blood flow to the brain. The patient is usually not aware of a change in his heart beat before the faint. During the period of unconsciousness, the patient may have a convulsion, again due to inadequate blood flow to the brain.

These problems with the heart's pacemaker or with the conducting wires usually occur in people who have atherosclerotic heart disease. Rarer instances concern people who have had heart disease due to diphtheria or other infections of the heart (myocarditis), rheumatic heart disease, or some forms of congenital heart disease (heart defects that children are born with). A complete heart block can occur as a complication of an acute heart attack or, as in Susan's case, can develop several years later.

The treatment of this condition is based primarily upon its recognition. The day that Susan fainted, she should have realized that something was seriously wrong, but she indulged herself in wishful thinking, or the ostrich game. "If I don't think about it, maybe it will go away." Of course, every person who faints does not have a heart block. Some people faint at the sight of blood or with pain or sudden fright. This involves another mechanism and is harmless unless the person hurts himself when he falls. But if a person who is over 35 or 40, and who is feeling fine, suddenly faints, this is probably a serious symptom.

Once the condition is recognized, the treatment is to replace the heart's electrical circuits with a mechanical device as soon as possible. Some degree of haste is in order because there is no way to predict when the next heart stoppage will occur, and the next episode may be the last.

The device used is called a pacemaker. Many misconceptions exist concerning them. The most common one is that the pacemaker is an artificial heart. It is not. It does not pump blood, nor does it prevent a person from having another heart attack or from dying of heart disease in another form. A pacemaker is an electronic unit with its own power supply (battery) connected to a wire (or wires) that are attached to the inside or the outside of the heart. The pacemaker regularly supplies an impulse that is carried by the wires to the heart muscle, where the impulse stimulates the heart to beat. If the heart is too weak from disease to contract, the pacemaker will not cause a heartbeat to be produced.

Some forms of pacemakers beat constantly and other forms operate only on demand. The latter form samples each of the heart's own beats and if one or more are missed, the pacemaker functions to supply the missing impulses as needed.

The pacemaker unit itself is usually placed within a pocket

just beneath the surface of the skin of the chest or abdomen. This location is chosen to facilitate replacement of the electronic unit or batteries. A wire runs from the pacemaker to the heart. The original method for establishing this connection was to perform chest surgery, opening the chest cage and sewing the end of the wire to the surface of the heart. A newer technique has been developed to avoid a major operation. The wire is threaded through a vein and directed to the interior of the heart. The wire is usually started in a vein in the neck or the shoulder. The progress of the wire is followed by a fluoroscope. When the tip of the wire reaches the interior of the heart, it is lodged in a corner of the right ventricle. The other end of the wire is connected to the pacemaker. The exposed piece of wire between the pacemaker and the neck vein is covered with skin, so that the entire system is beneath the body surface.

A great number of persons in the United States have pacemakers, and these patients are aware of the fact that at some point in time, they will have to have the unit changed. The pacemaker unit (batteries and electronic mechanism) are encased in a heavy plastic shell which protects the mechanism against body fluids. When the batteries are depleted, the entire unit must be changed.

Although the average pacemaker may have a lifespan of two years, many begin to fail at 18 months. Scientists have evaluated pacemaker function in many ways to try to predict when a failure is about to occur. The most reliable method of predicting battery exhaustion is still a change in the basic rate of the pacemaker unit, and patients are therefore instructed to periodically count their pulse rates. This may be helpful if the pacemaker is constantly functioning, but it becomes confusing when a demand pacemaker is in use. The demand pacemaker will not be functioning when the patient's heart rate is above a certain speed, so counting the pulse will give variable results depending upon whether the pacemaker is being called into function or whether the person's natural pacemaker is working at a faster rate.

This is the reason that, as patients near the end of the 18 month period, they must see their physician at increasingly frequent intervals. The physician can get an accurate count of the heart rate by placing a small magnet directly over the skin under which the pacemaker unit is implanted. The magnet disengages the demand function control, the pacemaker operates at its prescribed rate, and an electrocardiogram can then accurately record the pacer's rate. Some pacemakers are designed to speed up when the batteries near exhaustion, while others are designed to slow down. If the physician detects a change in rate, he may well advise changing the unit.

An instrument has been devised to enable a patient to check his pacemaker at home without journeying to the doctor's office. This will be very helpful to those people who live in rural areas and have to travel great distances to a pacemaker clinic. The function of this transtelephonic system was recently described by Drs. Pennock, Dreifus, Morse, and Watanbe of Hahnemann Hospital in Philadelphia. The patient is given a briefcase-sized transmitter to take home with him. Once a month, or at whatever interval is considered necessary, he places a telephone call to the pacemaker clinic. He then turns the transmitter on and holds in his hands two devices attached by wires to the transmitter. One handheld instrument is a magnet, which he places over his pacemaker. This converts his pacemaker to a steady output state and also detects the discharges of the pacemaker. The second wire is attached to a pulse detector which he slips over his index finger. The pulse detector signals each surge of blood which courses through the finger a fraction of a second after each heartbeat. The mouthpiece of the telephone is placed over a hole in his transmitter, and signals from each of the handheld electrodes are transmitted to the clinic. The technician at the clinic then activates a recording device which collects the information transmitted by the patient, and within a minute or so, enough data has been transcribed for later analysis.

Two types of information can be obtained from this transtelephonic system: the exact rate of the pacemaker and the capture of the heart. Each signal sent out by the pacer should be followed by a pulse at the fingertip. If one or more pacer signals are not followed by a pulse, then there is either a malfunction of the pacer or a crack in one of the wires leading from the pacing unit to the heart. If any abnormal function is determined, the clinic contacts the patient's personal physician, who then decides if replacement of the unit is advisable.

One of the drawbacks of this system is the expense of having a transmitter in each patient's home. An alternative approach would be for transmitters to be available at central points for patients to use collectively.

At times, a person who initially required a demand pacemaker may be able to have a fixed rate pacemaker installed when the first unit wears out. A demand pacer is used by those people who have only intermittent lapses of their natural pacemaker with variable periods when a mechanical pacemaker is not required. A fixed rate pacemaker operates continuously. The demand pacemaker functions only when a pause due to the slowing or stoppage of the natural pacemaker occurs in the normal heart rate. The demand pacemaker is preferred when dealing with intermittent lapses because its use avoids a competition between two pacer systems (the electronic unit and the heart's own pacemaker) and such competition could result in abnormally fast or irregular heart contraction. Many of the conditions requiring pacemaker implantation become worse with the passage of time, and ultimately the natural pacemaker completely ceases to function. When this event occurs, the demand unit is no longer necessary, and a fixed rate unit can be used. Advantages of the fixed rate units are that they cost less and often last longer than demand pacers. This latter point doesn't seem logical—why should a unit that is functioning part of the time wear out faster than a unit which functions constantly? Even though the demand unit is not triggering each heart beat, it is operating to detect every heart beat, so that it will know when to start discharging, and this standby activity requires battery energy.

The French have invented an atomic-powered pacemaker which has a probable life expectancy of ten years, but the cost of these units is prohibitive. The Cordis Company has devised a partial solution to the problem of battery life versus cost. They have developed a demand pacemaker that can operate on from 10 to 15 percent of the battery requirements of the older pacemakers. After it has been implanted in the body, the milliamperage output of this unit can be adjusted upwards or downwards. In this way, the physician can decrease the battery drain to the lowest level necessary to pace the patient after the operation is complete. At any later date, the amperage can be increased or decreased. The lifespan of this new unit is estimated to be between three and five years, although experience may reveal an even longer life.

7
Heart Failure

John was a 50-year-old insurance broker. He had been hospitalized three years ago with a heart attack. It had been a frightening experience for him, but he had survived and after three months had been able gradually to resume work. Initially he had lost the 30 pounds of weight as his doctor had advised. He had also given up smoking and held his work down to 30 hours a week. As time wore on, though, he gradually ate more, exercised less, and slipped back into the cigarette habit. He was also grinding out 55 hours a week on the job. But after all, he had two children in college and no one else was going to pay their bills.

He was more fatigued than usual and found himself stopping every few blocks to catch his breath when he was walking back to the office from lunch. "I'll have to start eating lunch in that restaurant around the corner. I hate the food, but it's not as far to walk." In the evenings before going to bed he noticed that the elastic bands of his socks were leaving imprints on his lower legs, and his ankles were indented by the top edges of his shoes. As he undid his belt, he felt relief; his abdomen appeared slightly swollen and a vague discomfort in his upper abdomen was lessened without his tight pants.

His wife Janet noted how tired he looked and reminded him that he had skipped his four-month checkup with his doctor. John promised to make another appointment soon, but he was just too busy this week to go. That night he fell asleep quickly, but about two a.m. he awoke feeling as though he needed more air. He got out of bed, went to the bathroom, and noted that lately he seemed to be getting up more at night to urinate. Last night it was three times, as a matter of fact. He went back to bed and after a while fell asleep again.

Three nights later John awoke at two a.m. horrified. He was suffocating! He couldn't get enough air. He was panting for breath and was making gurgling sounds in his chest. He awakened Janet and told her to call the doctor. John went to the window and threw it open to get more air. He felt a tightness developing in his chest similar to the one he experienced when he had his original heart attack. He went to the bedside table and found the nitroglycerine that his doctor had insisted he have. After a tablet dissolved under his tongue, the chest tightness was relieved, but the shortness of breath persisted. The doctor told Janet that he would meet them at the hospital emergency room.

His diagnosis was congestive heart failure with pulmonary edema. He had had warning signs of heart failure for days before the ultimate episode of pulmonary edema with fluid filling his lungs, but he had not recognized the impending danger.

Heart failure does not mean that the heart has stopped beating, and it does not mean that a person is having a heart attack or a myocardial infarction. It does mean that for a significant period of time the heart is not pumping enough blood. Heart failure may develop suddenly or gradually. It may occur immediately after a myocardial infarction or months or years later. The late development of heart failure is usually the result of the patient's placing greater demands on his heart over a period of time than the heart is able to tolerate. In mechanical terms, the heart is able to run nicely at 30 miles an hour, but the patient keeps racing it at 60. Heart failure may also occur in other forms of heart disease besides the type associated with atherosclerosis and myocardial infarction, if the heart is overworked.

A knowledge of some of the basic mechanisms involved in heart failure will help a person who has this problem to cope with the situation. The following is an explanation of some of the more important mechanisms.

The heart pumps a certain amount of blood per minute to the body. This amount of blood is called the cardiac output. The cardiac output for an average size man is five to six liters (quarts) per minute when he is awake but not active. This can be increased in the normal person to 30 or 35 liters per minute with exercise. After a heart attack, the heart muscle is weakened and the cardiac output *may* fall, transiently or permanently, to two to three liters per minute at rest. If the cardiac output falls below a certain level, the body will not receive adequate blood flow and a state of heart failure will be present. This is made most dramatically evident by an abnormal collection of fluid in the body. Let us see how this fluid accumulation occurs.

Many people are surprised to learn that the human body is 65 percent fluid. Each individual body cell contains fluid, and fluid circulates around each cell. A small amount of the body fluid circulates in the blood vessels as blood. Sodium (salt) and potassium are two of the most important ingredients in body fluids. Sodium is found primarily outside of the body cells, and potassium is located within the cells. The body regulates its own fluid volume by adjusting the amount of sodium and water that is excreted by the kidneys as urine. If we drink an excess of water, the kidneys eliminate the excess to reestablish normal body content. If we eat excess salt, the kidneys get rid of the unneeded amount. If we are dehydrated, the kidneys conserve water.

About 25 percent of the blood that the heart pumps is directed to the kidneys. From this large volume of blood the kidneys are constantly filtering out waste products and producing differing quantities of urine to adjust total body fluids.

If the blood flow to the kidneys is reduced, they will not function properly. Reduced blood flow could occur, for example, if the person were injured and had lost a lot of blood. The body attempts to make adjustments by the following mechanism. Kidney blood flow is monitored by special cells inside the arteries that feed the kidneys. If the flow falls below normal, these cells produce a substance which is released into the blood stream and eventually reaches the adrenal glands. The adrenal glands are triggered to produce certain hormones (aldosterone and cortisone) which are also released into the blood and eventually reach the kidneys again. Here the hormones "tell" the kidneys to conserve water and salt and therefore to reduce the volume of urine produced. The retained water and salt effectively increase the volume of blood contained in the blood vessel system (by expansion of the plasma, or fluid portion of the blood.) The result is an increase in the amount of blood reaching the kidneys, and these organs are again able to function.

The sensors that detect decreased kidney blood flow cannot differentiate between reduced flow caused by blood loss and reduced flow caused by poor heart function. In the latter case, the same protective mechanism operates. As a result, in the case of heart failure, an unnecessary increase in blood volume occurs.

The excess blood inside the blood vessels is detected by the heart, which temporarily works harder to move the blood along. However, the weakened heart cannot respond beyond a certain point, and the result is a buildup of back pressure and engorgement of the blood vessels.

The fluid portion of the blood (plasma) is constantly leaving the blood vessels and reentering them in the normal state of body operation. The purpose of this movement of fluid is to bathe the body cells in needed water, chemicals, and foods. As the plasma reenters the blood vessels, it brings with it wastes from the cells which are eventually carried to the kidneys. This movement of fluid to and from the blood vessels is controlled by pressures inside the vessels and in the body tissue spaces. In heart failure, when the kidney mechanism described above results in increased blood volume and pressure, the net effect is that it is easier for fluid to leave the vessels than it is for it to return. As a consequence, excess fluid (edema) surrounds the body cells.

A person in heart failure may accumulate as little as two or three pounds of excess fluid or, if the process has persisted for a long time, as much as 20 or 30 pounds. The fluid obeys the law of gravity, and if the person in heart failure is sitting in a chair much of the time, the edema will accumulate in his feet, ankles, and legs; if lying in bed on his back, it will tend to accumulate in the back and buttocks. The presence of edema can be detected by pressing into a soft area of tissue (as behind the ankle) with a finger. If the pressure is maintained for a minute or two, and then the finger is removed, a pit or depression will persist in the tissue where pressure was applied. The accumulation of fluid can also be surmised if a patient is weighed daily and if the weight is found to creep upward by a pound or two each day.

All persons with edema do not have heart failure. A small amount of edema may be present in the feet or ankles of persons with normal hearts who have been sitting or standing for long periods of time, as is the case when traveling in a car or working as a sales person who stands up for hours at a time. Diseases of the kidneys themselves and some forms of liver disease will also cause edema.

The person with heart failure and edema who has been standing or sitting much of the day may experience a strange development known as nocturnal dyspnea (night-shortness of breath) when he lies down in bed at the end of the day. The fluid which has accumulated in the legs and feet is no longer held there by gravity, and the excess fluid gradually returns to the blood stream and overloads the circulation. Pressure rises in the blood vessels and starts to force excess amounts of plasma out of the small blood vessels (capillaries) into the tissue. The lungs, which were previously protected by gravity and their high location in the body when the person was erect, are now affected. The plasma oozes from the capillaries into the tiny air spaces in the lungs and blocks off the gas exchange that normally occurs there. If the person is still awake as this is happening, he may notice a gradually increasing shortness of breath and find that if he raises his head and shoulders higher by propping himself up on pillows, he is more comfortable. If asleep at this time, he may instead suddenly awaken and find himself gasping for breath.

The normal reaction in this instance is to sit up or get out of bed and walk around, which again throws gravity into the situation and helps to correct the situation temporarily by drawing the excess fluid back down to the legs. Another medical term for this congestion of the lungs is pulmonary edema (pulmonary = lungs).

Pulmonary edema may occur in another circumstance in heart failure. The heart is basically a double pump. The right side of the heart receives blood from the body via the veins and pumps the blood through the lungs to receive oxygen. The left side of the heart now receives this blood from the lungs and pumps it back to the body. The left side of the heart has more work to do and is therefore equipped with larger muscles which contain the majority of the blood vessels that feed the heart (coronary arteries). In the event of a myocardial infarction, therefore, the left side is usually more severely, or exclusively, injured. The result is that one pump is now weaker than it should be. The right side of the heart will still be able to pump a normal amount of blood into the lungs, but the left side may not be able to accept the total volume and return it to the body. As a result, the blood vessels of the lungs become abnormally engorged, and the increased pressure inside the vessels can force plasma through the walls of the capillaries into the air spaces of the lungs.

This explains why some people have mild pulmonary edema in the early stages of a myocardial infarct or even with severe angina, in which case the left side of the heart is suffering from a lack of coronary blood flow and may be weakened. This also is the mechanism involved when a person with a weakened heart experiences shortness of breath when he is exercising (such as walking.) If this person stops exercising, or slows down, the left side of the heart is able to catch up to its task and remove the excess blood (and pressure) from the lungs.

A less dramatic consequence of this imbalance between the two pumps is seen when back pressure rises in the lungs gradually but not to the point where plasma oozes into the air spaces. This elevated pressure in the blood vessels of the lungs requires increased work from the right pump. It must work harder to get blood into these blood vessels which are already filled with blood. In time, this circumstance tires the right side of the heart, and it is unable to pump a normal volume of blood. In turn, this produces a backing up of blood in the veins that normally drain into the right pump. One result of this is that the liver, located in the right upper part of the abdomen and richly supplied with blood vessels, becomes filled with blood. This causes a swelling of the liver that the patient may recognize as a sense of fullness and heaviness or soreness in the upper abdomen. The back pressure phenomenon extends to all the other parts of the body and can interfere with the normal function of organs. Back pressure also tends to aggravate the production of general body edema.

The treatment of this problem involves many factors. In general, the person's activities are reduced to decrease the demands that are placed on the heart. If the situation is severe, or if there is shortness of breath, oxygen is used. This gives some relief from the lack of air and results in an increased delivery of oxygen to the body cells which may be in short supply. Salt is restricted in the diet, because any additional accumulation of fluid in the body must be accompanied by a certain amount of salt, to maintain the usual water-to-salt ratio. In some instances, water and other fluids will be restricted until the situation improves. If the person is anxious, some form of sedation is prescribed, because the more agitated a person is, the harder the heart works as a result of the release of adrenaline from the adrenal glands. Digitalis in one form or another is usually used to treat heart failure. This drug slows excessively fast heart rates and strengthens the force of each heart contraction. Finally, some form of a diuretic is usually employed. These drugs affect the kidneys and cause them to increase the formation of urine with the resultant loss of excess fluid and salt that has accumulated.

8

Tachycardia—
Rapid Heart Rhythms

Abnormal heart speeds and rhythms can occur in normal persons as well as in those who have various types of heart disease. Some rhythms are harmless, but others may tire the heart by causing it to overwork. As stated before, the normal heart rate is 60 to 100 beats per minute. An average person has a rate of 70 to 80. During exercise, excitement, or when a person is running a fever, the heart rate may increase to 120 to 130 beats per minute. This acceleration is perfectly normal.

Some persons are very much aware of an accelerated pulse when they are excited or nervous. Such a person may believe that something is wrong with his heart because he can feel it beating. If he is able to count his pulse, however, and if it is in the range described above, he should realize that there is usually nothing wrong with the heart itself.

The pulse is counted by placing the tip of the index finger of one hand on the opposite wrist at the side of the wrist that the thumb arises from. Cords will be felt running along under the skin, and between these cords a pulsation is felt. If the index finger is pressed too hard, the pulse will be obliterated, and if pressure is too light, no pulse will be felt. To determine the pulse or heart rate, count the number of impulses felt during one minute.

The commonest disturbance of the normal heart beat is premature beats (extrasystoles). The patient may sense this as a skip in the pulse or as a thump in the chest or even as a feeling that the heart is turning over. The fact is that a beat is occurring earlier than expected. The beat is felt as a weak or soft impulse if one is checking the pulse at this time. This is because the heart did not have sufficient time to fill properly after the preceding beat and not as much blood was ejected with the early beat. The next heart contraction is usually stronger than normal, since there is a pause after the early beat, and the heart fills with more blood than usual and ejects a larger volume of blood for this single beat. Thus the heart does not actually pause or skip a beat, and the thump felt in the chest is due to a more forceful beat that vibrates the chest. These premature beats interfere very little with normal heart function unless they occur many times a minute or unless the heart is very weak—as it is following a myocardial infarction.

Premature beats occur in normal persons. They are more likely to occur if the person is fatigued or has overstimulated himself with nicotine or coffee.

After a myocardial infarction, these early beats assume a different significance. In this situation the heart is injured and is irritable ("sore as a boil"). Abnormal and fast heart rhythms are prone to occur, and early beats may trigger them. By analyzing the electrocardiographic appearance of such beats, the physician can often predict whether or not they are potentially serious and can then use various drugs to block the trigger.

The next most common disturbance of cardiac rhythm seen in persons with atherosclerotic heart disease is atrial flutter and atrial fibrillation. The right and left atria are thin-walled chambers that receive blood from the body and lungs. The ventricles of the heart, which are the main pumping chambers that send blood to the body and lungs, are filled from these reservoirs—the atria. Normally, each heart beat consists of a contraction of the right and left atria, followed in $^{2}\!\%_{00}$ of a second by the right and left ventricles after they have filled with blood from the atria. The impulse that signals these events to occur spreads from the sino-atrial node (the pacemaker) through the atria and then down to the ventricles. The timing of the contraction of the various parts of the heart is caused by the method by which this impulse spreads throughout the heart.

The S-A node usually initiates the heartbeat. At times, other areas of the heart may take over temporarily as the pacemaker. This is similar to the situation in life where the parents are normally the guiding hands that influence their children. In certain circumstances, other people, such as close friends, may come to exert a stronger influence on the behavior of the children than the parents. In atrial flutter and fibrillation, other areas of the atria take command of the heartbeat away from the normal pacemaker. This may occur because the S-A node is not getting sufficient blood to function properly or because there is disease in the tissue of the heart where it is located. Certain drugs can also suppress the normal pacemaker and allow another part of the heart to assume control over heartbeat. With atrial flutter or fibrillation, the atria are induced to beat so rapidly that they are actually quivering. They are unable then to propel blood actively into the ventricles, and the latter fill passively. Instead of being forcibly propelled into the ventricles, the blood just runs down from the atria to the ventricles when the valves between these two chambers are open.

The ventricles ordinarily follow the atria and beat or contract each time that the atria are stimulated to beat. If this were allowed to happen with atrial flutter or fibrillation, the ventricles would be stimulated almost 300 times per minute, and they, too, would be quivering and would not be able to pump blood to the body and lungs. A protective mechanism, a governor, so to speak, exists along the nervous pathway that connects the atria and the ventricles. It will not allow 300 stimulations per minute to pass through it. When a series of stimuli as rapid as this enters this special tissue, it blocks the fast rate and allows only every second, third, or fourth impulse to travel on to the ventricles. This area of the heart is called the atrio-ventricular node (A-V node).

The principal practical difference between atrial flutter and atrial fibrillation is that, in atrial flutter, the A-V node allows every second or fourth beat to pass through to the ventricles in a regular, orderly fashion, so that the ventricles are beating at a regular speed. If the atria are contracting 300 times a minute, and the A-V node allows every second impulse to pass, then the ventricles will beat 150 times per minute. If, on the other hand, the A-V node allows every fourth beat to pass, the ventricles will beat 75 times per minute. This rate is within the normal range of the heart beat and would not be associated with any cardiac dysfunction. In atrial fibrillation, however, the A-V node allows a variable number of impulses to pass down to the ventricles so that the ventricles are not beating regularly. There is an unsteady rhythm. Several faster beats may be followed by beats spaced further apart.

Fibrillation impairs the efficiency of the ventricles as pumps, and they do not pump as much blood as they would if the rhythm were regular. If the rate of the ventricles is about 90–100, the efficiency of the heart may be reduced only about 10 percent. If, on the other hand, the rate speeds up to 130 or 140 beats per minute, cardiac efficiency may be reduced 40–50 percent. A rapid atrial fibrillation is a common precipitating cause of heart failure.

Atrial fibrillation or atrial flutter may occur intermittently. In other words, a person may have a normal heartbeat, then develop abnormal rhythms for minutes or hours, and then spontaneously change back to a normal rhythm. During the episode of abnormal heartbeat, the person may be aware of a rapid beating of the pulse or an irregularity of the heartbeat. This may be associated with no other symptoms, or he may experience a feeling of apprehension, weakness, or shortness of breath. If the person suffers from angina pectoris, an episode of atrial flutter or fibrillation may induce an attack of angina with its resulting chest pain.

When these abnormal rhythms are occurring intermittently, it may be hard for the person to describe to his doctor later exactly what happened. If his heart is beating normally during his visit to the doctor's office, the physician will not be able to make an exact diagnosis. The patient, in this situation, can help establish the correct diagnosis if he can count his pulse rate and notice whether the pulse seems to be regular or irregular during an attack. The other alternative is to try to have an electrocardiogram taken during an episode. The diagnosis is definitely established by a typical appearance on the ECG.

Various drugs, digitalis, quinidine, Pronestyl®, and propanolol—are used to control these rhythms. If the ventricles are beating too rapidly, the heart rate is first slowed, and then conversion to a regular heart rhythm is attempted. An electrical shock applied to the chest (defibrillation) is sometimes used to change the rhythms back to normal. This maneuver is used if drug control is unsuccessful or if it is important to change the rhythm back to normal rapidly. Drug conversion can sometimes take days, while the electrical method is accomplished in minutes. Electrical conversion, or defibrillation, is usually performed in a hospital and is preceded by a light anesthesia to avoid discomfort for the patient.

There is another problem associated with atrial fibrillation —thromboembolism, or blood clots. Each atrium has a small appendage shaped like a dog's ear. This is called the auricle. This small pocket is connected to the interior of each atrium. When the atria fibrillate, there is no general contraction of the chamber to empty the blood. Blood tends to become trapped in the auricles, and it may actually clot. In a small percentage of persons with atrial fibrillation these small clots form, and part of the clot may break away and get swept into the circulation. If the clot originated in the right auricle, it gets trapped in the lungs as an embolus. If the clot originated in the left auricle, it can travel to any part of the general circulation and finally rest in one of the body organs such as the brain, spleen, kidney, or an extremity.

The blood clot, or embolus, may or may not completely obstruct the blood vessel that finally traps it. It may or may not cause death of tissue in the organ that it finally rests in, depending on whether or not other blood vessels (collateral vessels) can adequately supply blood to the involved area. Such an embolus usually does cause tissue death in the brain, and this is *one* of the causes of strokes. This circumstance, the release of clots from an auricle, can occur when the heart is going from a regular rhythm to fibrillation and back again, or during constant fibrillation. The probable course of events is that during fibrillation the clot is formed. When the heart reverts to a regular rhythm, the contraction of the formerly quivering atrium actually pushes the clot out of the side pocket into the general flow of blood to be swept away. If this embolus situation occurs, the usual therapeutic attack is to prescribe anticoagulant drugs for the patient. These drugs do not prevent blood coagulation, but they do make it more difficult for blood clots to occur. The drug may therefore decrease the likelihood of an embolus.

In some cases, and in particular after repeated episodes of slipping back and forth into fibrillation, the heart cannot be converted to a normal rhythm and the patient continues to fibrillate for the balance of his life. This is not as bad as it sounds, since drugs can control the speed of fibrillation. The heart efficiency may be decreased by a factor of only ten percent, which most patients can tolerate without difficulty. After a time, most people adjust to the situation and are not aware of an irregular pulse unless they exercise and increase the heart rate.

A final category of tachycardias includes atrial tachycardia, nodal tachycardia, supraventricular tachycardia, and ventricular tachycardia. These are all regular, fast rhythms. They may occur in healthy persons, although some types occur most often in people with heart disease. The patient usually feels a rapid heartbeat and some degree of chest awareness or discomfort. If the rate is very fast, adequate blood may not be supplied to the brain and the patient may lose consciousness. These tachycardias may stop by themselves or they may require a physician's attention and special drugs to convert them to a normal rhythm. In general, the same drugs used to treat atrial fibrillation and atrial flutter are used for these rhythms, and electrical conversion may also be used. The identification of the specific type of disorder involved is important because ventricular tachycardia has an affinity for changing into ventricular fibrillation. This is a grave disorder in which the ventricles quiver instead of beating, and very little blood is pumped from the ventricles. The patient with ventricular fibrillation usually loses consciousness within 15–30 seconds after the onset of the disorder, and if it is not terminated spontaneously or by forms of treatment, death will occur within five minutes.

Ventricular fibrillation is most likely to occur soon after a myocardial infarction, and this is one of the chief reasons for putting this type of patient in a special coronary care unit where equipment is at hand to treat the problem immediately. The usual form of treatment is to apply an electrical shock (defibrillation) to the chest over the heart. If the electrical current is applied quickly, it usually improves the heart rhythm. Cardiopulmonary resuscitation (artificial respiration and heart massage) can also be utilized at this time to help the patient.

The important thing to remember about tachycardias is that treatment is available to handle them. The patient should seek medical assistance either to get reassurance if the problem turns out to be of no consequence, or to receive treatment if the situation warrants it. A grown man or woman who faints for no apparent reason and does not seek medical attention is flirting with danger and maybe death.

9
What Are These Pills For?

If you are taking medicine that your doctor has prescribed for a heart condition, you should know the names of the pills and their dosage. It is also helpful to be able to recognize their appearance. The reason for this is that some day you may require the attention of a doctor who has never seen you before. If you are on your summer vacation hundreds of miles away from home and develop strange symptoms that might represent an allergy or overdose of one of your medicines, the physician will have to know which drugs you are taking in order to treat you properly. If you do not have the pills with you, or if you do not have the pill container that has the name of the drug written on it, it will be impossible to tell the new doctor what drugs you are taking. If the doctor is unable to get in touch with your own physician or druggist, this important information might remain unknown. Even if you have your pills, it might be impossible for him to distinguish between the hundreds or thousands of small, round, white pills that exist. A more common circumstance in which you might need to know the names of your pills would be if you were traveling and happened to lose your medicine. At this time a visit to a local physician with the report of this fact, the exact names and doses of your medicine, and the frequency that you take them would enable him to replace your drugs with a minimum of inconvenience to you.

You should also know, in general, what these pills are supposed to be doing for you, and you should know what side effects they could produce. It is important to be able to differentiate between side effects and symptoms of disease. If the symptoms are not recognized for what they really are, they may eventually develop into serious and even life-threatening forms of disease.

The following is a résumé of some of the more commonly used cardiac drugs, their principal actions, side effects, and dangers.

Digitalis. Commonly used digitalis preparations are digitalis leaf, digoxin (Lanoxin®), digitoxin (Crystodigin®), and gitaligin. This family of drugs is used to treat and prevent heart failure and various types of rapid heartbeat. It operates by producing a more forceful contraction of the heart, and by regulating the speed of transmission of impulses through the heart's conduction system (electrical system).

The person taking digitalis usually recalls the events that led to the initial use of the drug. The episode may have begun by marked shortness of breath or swelling of the legs and ankles, or by a sensation of palpitation in the chest. After the initial problem had been controlled, the doctor told the patient to continue taking the same medicine to prevent a recurrence of symptoms. In time, some patients gain a false sense of security from their good health, and without consulting their physician, stop taking their digitalis drugs. This is a very unwise and dangerous expression of independence. The drug should be started and stopped only on the order of a physician.

When a digitalis drug is first used, the patient may take two, three, or four pills a day for several days, and then the dose is usually decreased to one or two pills a day for the duration of their use. Over months or years, it may be necessary to make minor adjustments in the dosage, taking one extra pill a week or decreasing the dose to one smaller size tablet to be taken daily. The goal is to maintain an adequate amount of the drug in the body to do the job it was prescribed for. Too much of the drug will cause symptoms of an overdose, and too little will not accomplish the objective. The body destroys or excretes a certain amount of the drug each day. The doctor's job is to determine by physical examination, and at times by certain tests, that the amount of the drug taken daily is replacing the amount lost by the body. This "fine tuning" of the digitalis dosage can be performed only by your physician.

A common sight in hospital emergency rooms is the patient who has poisoned himself with digitalis. The usual story is that, whenever he felt unusually short of breath or had chest pains, he took extra digitalis to stimulate his heart. This patient would be horrified if you suggested to him that he play Russian roulette with a loaded revolver, but he has been doing essentially the same thing with his digitalis. The following story illustrates the problem.

Henry was a 70-year-old fisherman who had been my patient for five years. He had angina pectoris in addition to skin cancers that kept cropping out on his ears and the backs of his hands after 60 years of skin punishment from the sun. In the fourth year of treatment he developed atrial fibrillation for the first time, but we were able to control it adequately with digoxin. He took one tablet a day. Ten months later, Henry came into the office complaining about his heart jumping around more than usual. After an examination and an electrocardiogram, we found that his heart was fibrillating again. His dose of digoxin was increased temporarily but this time his heart did not revert to a regular rhythm. Quinidine was added to his list of medicines in an attempt to correct things. Then Henry began to lose weight. When we questioned him about this, he said that he had put himself on a diet, and we accepted this reason for the loss of weight. Almost two months after this he fainted at home after returning from an all-day fishing trip. He was brought to the emergency room at the hospital, and on examination, it was found that his heart was beating very rapidly and that his blood pressure was below normal.

After repeated questioning, we finally found what was wrong. When Henry was first given the digoxin pills, he found he was feeling much better. But after that time, whenever he felt tired or had an angina pain not immediately relieved by nitroglycerine he would take an extra digoxin pill. Whenever asked about the dose he was taking, he would say that he was taking one a day. He was actually taking several pills a day. The result was that he gradually built up too much digoxin in his body. An excess of digoxin can cause the heart to fibrillate—the very condition that it was prescribed to reduce in the first place. When we found that he was in atrial fibrillation two months previous, our first move was to increase his digoxin dosage. The "diet" that Henry put himself on was actually a loss of appetite that is one of the early symptoms of too much digoxin. When the truth was finally revealed, we stopped his digoxin for four days and the symptoms disappeared. Henry learned his lesson this time.

An overdose of digitalis can develop gradually over a period of weeks or may occur rather suddenly in a few days. The sudden overdose may occur during the course of an illness such as diarrhea or vomiting, which dehydrates the patient. The commonest symptom of excess digitalis is a loss of appetite or even vomiting. The patient may feel a general sense of poor health or may notice that his pulse has either slowed down dramatically or has become much more rapid or irregular. A change in vision is another important sign of excess digitalis. The patient may notice over several days or weeks that his eyesight has become markedly diminished or that strange lights or colors are developing in his field of vision.

Digitalis is used to treat heart failure, but an excess of digitalis *may result in heart failure.* The patient may again develop the very symptoms for which he was originally treated. This puzzling situation is very deceiving to the person who tries to manipulate his own dose of medicine according to the way he is currently feeling. When the doctor diagnoses this problem, the dose of digitalis is reduced, and usually within a few days the symptoms disappear.

Pronestyl and Quinidine. Pronestyl and quinidine are most often prescribed for the treatment of irregular heart rhythms, various types of rapid heart rhythms, or frequent premature beats (extrasystoles). Pronestyl and quinidine are rapidly eliminated from the body, and a dose exerts its effect for only four to six hours. Quinidex®, Quinaglute®, and Cardioquin® have a longer lasting effect, eight to twelve hours. It is easy to see that the drugs must be taken on a regular schedule throughout the 24 hours of the day if the desired effect is to be achieved.

In some cases, when the underlying problem is one of a rapid heartbeat of minor consequence, the patient may be told to take a certain number of pills on a regular schedule only when the disturbance is noticed. When a normal heartbeat is resumed, the patient discontinues the medicine until the next episode. The decision whether treatment with these medicines should be continuous or intermittent should rest, of course, with the physician.

People have a variable tolerance for these drugs. One person may be able to take eight pills a day without unusual symptoms, whereas half that dose may produce diarrhea in another person. A loss of appetite, nausea, and diarrhea are the commonest signs of an overdose or intolerance. An excessive amount may produce a drop in blood pressure with symptoms of weakness, dizziness, or even fainting. A change in the normal speed and rhythm of the heartbeat would also make your physician suspicious of possible overdose or unusual susceptibility. Various types of skin rash may be the first sign of allergy to this family of drugs, and the appearance of any skin rash is a reason for the patient to consult his doctor.

Anticoagulants. Anticoagulants are used to attempt to prevent or delay the formation of blood clots within blood vessels in various parts of the body. They are prescribed for some patients who have angina pectoris, a previous myocardial infarct or stroke, atrial fibrillation with embolus, or thrombophlebitis with lung embolism, or when symptoms are present suggesting inadequate blood flow to the heart, brain, or legs. Some patients with artificial heart valves also take these drugs to prevent blood clots from forming in the valves. Many factors determine whether or not anticoagulants should be used in a particular case, and the decision to use them must rest with the physician.

Some commonly used anticoagulants in pill form are Dicumarol®, Coumadin®, Panwarfin®, Sintrom®, and Liquamar®. Under certain circumstances, patients may be given anticoagulants by injection. Heparin is the most frequently used drug in this category.

The use of anticoagulants requires that the patient's blood be tested periodically to determine whether the dosage is adequate or excessive. Many variables affect the amount of drug required. For example, bacteria that are normally present in the intestinal tract produce vitamin K, which counteracts the effect of such drugs as Dicumarol. If the patient takes an antibiotic for some unrelated reason, such as for an infected tooth, the antibiotic may decrease the number of bacteria producing vitamin K. The same dose of Dicumarol may produce an unusual degree of anticoagulation. Certain types of foods may counteract the effect of the drugs. For unknown reasons, when some people travel from one part of the country to another, their anticoagulation mechanism may be altered and a change in drug dosage may be necessary. Many drugs will also alter the effectiveness of the oral anticoagulants. This is particularly true of certain sleeping pills and aspirin (salicylates). The dose of anticoagulant can be adjusted if the same amount of sleeping pill or aspirin is taken every day, but varying the amount from day to day cannot be compensated for. A list of drugs that work counter to the oral anticoagulants is not included here because additional drugs are being constantly discovered. Your physician should be your guide.

The prothrombin time is the commonly used blood test to determine the effect of anticoagulants. Some patients demonstrate a remarkably constant prothrombin time over a period of months or years, but this does not alter the necessity for periodic blood tests to determine the exact action of the drug. A certain number of patients taking anticoagulants develop severe bleeding complications that may even result in their death. It is not a surprise to physicians that many unfortunate people who have fatal bleeding complications did not follow their doctor's advice by taking periodic blood tests.

Usually the development of an abnormal degree of anticoagulation will produce symptoms that the patient can recognize. Every patient taking these drugs should look at his skin after bathing to see if any bruises or small hemorrhages have developed. A bruise after minimal injury or spontaneous bruising is frequently the first sign of difficulty. A second common sign is the appearance of blood in the urine. Therefore, the color of the urine should be noted. Bleeding into the intestinal tract is another sign of difficulty, and blood in the stool will be either red or black as tar. With the development of any of these signs, the patient should stop taking the drug and get in touch with his doctor. Depending upon the severity of the bleeding and the patient's prothrombin time, as well as his basic problem, the physician may prescribe an antidote or just withhold the drug for several days.

In the event that the person taking anticoagulant drugs is injured, and particularly if the skin is cut or torn, bleeding may be excessive. Most cases of bleeding can be controlled satisfactorily by applying firm pressure over the laceration. This stops the blood flow, and clotting will usually occur, but at a slower speed than normal.

Diuretics. A great many drugs have been developed to promote the excretion of salt and walter through the kidneys. Diuril®, HydroDIURIL®, Enduron®, hydrochlorothiazide, Exna®, Renese®, Lasix®, Esidrix®, Dyrenium®, Dyazide®, Aldactone®, Aldactazide®, and Naqua® are just some of the names that are found in this family of drugs. Patients frequently use the terms "water pills," "piddling pills," and "dehydrating pills" to describe their action. They are used to treat congestive heart failure and hypertension.

Diuretics encourage the kidneys to increase the concentration of sodium excreted in the daily volume of urine. As the sodium excretion increases, so does water excretion, and the total daily volume of urine usually increases. The patient may recognize this phenomenon by an increase in the frequency of urination, especially at night.

Many such drugs also increase the loss of potassium from the body through the kidneys and urine (Aldactone and Dyrenium are exceptions to this). Potassium is a vital element found in all the cells of the body, and its loss as a result of diuretics is unintentional, representing a side effect. When body potassium levels fall too low, patients often develop muscle weakness. Potassium tends to counteract the action of digitalis, and if a potassium deficit develops, the patient may develop signs of digitalis excess.

Depending upon the individual case and the strength of the diuretic, the physician may prescribe extra potassium for the patient. This may be in the form of a medicine such as potassium chloride tablets, Kaon® liquid or tablets, Kao-chlor®, or K-Lyte®. Certain foods have a high potassium content, such as citrus fruits and juices, tomatoes and to-mato juice, and bananas, and these may be prescribed instead of medicinal potassium.

In some instances the diuretic agent may originally or subsequently prove to be too strong for the patient, in which case he may experience generalized weakness, a loss of strength, or fainting. These signs may also develop if the person loses an unusual amount of salt from the body as might occur with a siege of diarrhea or excessive perspiring in hot weather.

Like most drugs, diuretics may also produce various types of skin rash. They may also precipitate an attack of gout by raising the body content of uric acid, which causes gout. An early indication of gout is the development of a very sore joint. This usually disappears after the drug is discontinued or changed.

Some patients with diabetes may find that they require more insulin or a larger dose of their oral antidiabetic drugs, because in certain persons the diuretic agents raise the level of blood sugar.

Your physician may or may not want you to restrict your intake of salt while you are taking the diuretic. It is proper for you to question him about his exact wishes on this matter. The severity of your disease and the strength of the individual diuretic drug that you are using will determine the answer.

Nitroglycerine. This is very effective in stopping the pain of angina pectoris. Some preparations of nitroglycerine are swallowed, but usually a small white pill is placed under the tongue and allowed to dissolve. If the pain is relieved and then recurs, a second or third nitroglycerine pill may be taken. If the pills are taken too close together, the blood pressure may fall and the person will feel faint. This can be remedied by lying down until the effect of the drug wears off.

When the typical chest pain of angina begins, a pill should be taken. There is no advantage in waiting one, two, or five minutes. Some patients hesitate to use nitroglycerine because they fear that they will become addicted to it or that it will lose its effectiveness. If the pill does lose its effectiveness, it is usually because the disease in the coronary arteries has progressed beyond the point at which this type of medicine will help. The patient has not developed a tolerance to the drug, and addiction to nitroglycerine does not occur.

Probably the greatest usefulness of nitroglycerine is in its ingestion two or three minutes before beginning exercise or encountering a stressful situation, either of which may trigger angina pains. Many people with angina have more difficulty at the start of a particular activity than they have later on. For example, many people will have angina at the start of a two-mile walk rather than at the end. Similarly, a golfer will often feel the chest tightness on the first hole rather than on the eighteenth. Taking nitroglycerine at the beginning of the walk or at the beginning of the golf game can avert the attack.

Nitroglycerine is a very unstable drug. It is packed in a dark or opaque bottle to protect it from light. It is also very sensitive to heat, and a bottle of nitroglycerine left on a windowsill in the sunshine, or in the glove compartment of a car during the summer, will be quickly destroyed by the heat. The drug begins to deteriorate in the air once the manufacturer's seal has been broken. Pills kept in the original container should usually be discarded after six months. A nitroglycerine tablet carried loose in a coat pocket may lose its potency in two or three days. Tablets carried in pill boxes may deteriorate in from one to three weeks.

Many patients will notice a burning sensation inside their mouth when they place a nitroglycerine tablet under their tongue. The burning occurs at the site of contact between the pill and the mucous membrane of the mouth. Other patients note either a distinct throbbing in their head or a headache of variable intensity. If either of these symptoms usually occurs when the prescription is new and then gradually disappears, it may be a clue that the nitro tablets are losing their strength. If the symptoms reoccur when a fresh supply of nitroglycerine is purchased, then you have an accurate device to measure the life span of your medication.

Long Acting Nitrates. Many products available on the market are supposed to combine the effects of nitroglycerine with a much longer duration of action. These drugs are generally classified as coronary vasodilators. They may be in the form of layered pills or of capsules containing many small pellets The medicine is supposed to be slowly released in the intestinal tract and to have a reported duration of action of from six to twelve hours, depending upon the product.

A great deal of current medical opinion holds that these drugs are of limited value (if not completely useless). Once the active ingredients are absorbed through the intestinal tract, they are carried to the liver and changed into substances which are not capable of increasing the blood flow to the heart. Why then were these drugs prescribed? A logical question if you are paying the drug bill. The reason is that both patient and doctor have been under the impression that the drugs were accomplishing something beneficial. Actually, both parties have often fallen into a snare. Let's go back to the beginning and see how it happened.

These drugs are invariably prescribed for persons who have angina. One day you suddenly develop chest pains which come and go. It is naturally a frightening experience. You go to your doctor, or maybe to a heart specialist, and after a thorough examination, you are told that you have angina. The examination and the doctor's explanation give you confidence that you have a problem which can be controlled. If there are factors present which aggravate the angina, such as being overweight, smoking, extra tension, long working hours, nagging problems, then a solution is sought for each of these. In addition, the doctor prescribes a long-acting coronary vasodilator.

In a great many cases, the symptoms gradually subside. The patient continues to see his doctor periodically for check-ups and reassurance. Weight loss, abstinence from cigarette smoking, and the avoidance of tension-inducing situations continue along with regular pill-taking. But which one of these many factors was responsible for the control of the angina? Was it the weight loss, stopping cigarettes, the relaxation, the reassurance of the doctor, or taking the pills?

At any rate, a great many doctors have found that if they discontinue the use of these drugs, their patients do not suffer a reoccurrence of anginal pain. Further investigation is warranted on this matter, and a more positive answer should be available in the future regarding the true usefulness of this class of drugs.

Another class of anti-anginal medicine is taken by different means. Instead of swallowing a pill, a tablet is either dissolved in the mouth or chewed. Medication taken by this route (as is nitroglycerine), goes directly into the general body circulation without first passing through the liver. The liver therefore doesn't have a chance to inactivate the drug before it can reach its point of action. This class of drugs appears to be effective in controlling angina, but the duration of their effect may only be an hour or so.

10

Rehabilitation— The Road Back

You have been released from the hospital after your myocardial infarct. Your first three or four weeks there required very strict rest. As time passed you were allowed to feed yourself, go to the bathroom, bathe yourself, and finally walk around the room. This all progressed in gradual stages. You accepted this restricted activity because you understood that your heart needed rest and time to heal itself.

This time was also put to other good use. During those first days, besides guarding against complications and treating any that developed, your doctor was evaluating your total health situation. He was looking for aggravating factors that may have precipitated your heart attack. If you had been a cigarette smoker, during this period you refrained from smoking. After a three-week period of abstinence, you at least had a good head start to stay off the habit. You understood that it was vitally important to stop smoking in order to prevent further trouble. You were also told that you were overweight, and because of the strict diet that had been imposed upon you, you had already lost ten pounds of the 30 that you eventually had to peel off. If you had an under-lying problem with hypertension (high blood pressure), the doctors had a chance to start controlling that factor. Your blood cholesterol and other fats were analyzed, and any special diets were discussed with you and your family.

It was also helpful for your self-confidence to have the doctor examine you, after you had bathed yourself in the bathroom, and reassure you that your heart was functioning nicely after that exercise. That gave you less to worry about when you were home again. Your doctor also took advantage of his many visits with you to inquire into the usual daily activities that you performed prior to your heart attack. He knew what type of work you were accustomed to, what type of exercise you did or did not indulge in, and what your rest patterns were. The doctor had also talked with your wife to reassure her and give her instructions about your subsequent activities and diet.

During this time, your physician was also attempting to assess your psychological attitude toward your health problem as well as your wife's attitudes.

The doctor also had assured you that, since everything was going so nicely, you could probably return to your usual job. You would start work part time, but there was a good chance that you could go back to working 40 hours per week. You were able to tell your employer that you would be back in about six or eight more weeks, and that had satisfied him.

All of these factors are evaluated in the person who has had a myocardial infarct. The immediate problem, its diagnosis and treatment, the observation for complications, evaluation of predisposing factors, analysis of the social and psychological circumstances of the patient and his immediate family—all of these factors have a bearing on the patient's recovery.

You are told that it takes approximately six weeks for the heart to heal after an infarction. You are instructed to minimize your activity at home for another three weeks. You will be allowed to do approximately the same things at home that you were doing in the hospital before your discharge. Your doctor will see you periodically during this time to examine you and to be sure that your recovery is progressing on schedule.

After this six-week period (from the onset of the attack), your doctor will instruct you how gradually to increase your activity until you are back to the level that you were used to prior to your illness. Again, he will examine you at intervals to be sure that your heart is tolerating each new step. He will ask if you have any symptoms that might be distress signals from your heart, such as chest pain, shortness of breath, fatigue, or swelling of the ankles. He can tell many things about your heart function from your pulse, blood pressure, the sounds that come from your heart and lungs, and from any changes that occur after you do mild exercise in his office.

Despite all reassurances, it is normal for a person to have a certain amount of anxiety about himself after a heart attack. This is good to a certain extent and acts as a protective mechanism of the body. Overconcern, however, can greatly prolong the convalescence and can lead to an unnecessarily restricted life.

One common problem is the evaluation of any possible chest pain. The doctor has repeatedly asked you if you have any chest pain, and so you are watching for it. When we are in a state of normal health, we have many aches and pains in our bodies which we usually ignore. These pains have a new significance if they occur in the chest after a heart attack. Most patients do begin to notice a pain here or there. They have subconsciously focused their attention on this possibility. To help you sort out the important from the unimportant pains, you should be aware that pain from the heart (angina or another heart attack) will usually occur in the same location repeatedly. It will also, in general, have the same intensity or quality as the original pain that you suffered with the myocardial infarct. If distinguishing one pain from another becomes a problem, your doctor can frequently offer help by having you try nitroglycerine when the pains occur. In general, pain originating in the heart will be relieved by the nitroglycerine within one or two minutes, whereas other pain will either be unaffected or relieved five to ten minutes after taking the pill.

Another problem is deciding what is and what is not shortness of breath. Sighing, taking one or two deep breaths periodically, is frequently caused by anxiety and not by heart problems. Significant shortness of breath is more likely to occur when the patient is walking or climbing stairs than when he is sitting in a chair, reading a book, or watching television. Serious shortness of breath is likely to be accompanied by a fast pulse. A person lying flat on his back and complaining of shortness of breath usually does not have a serious problem either; if he did, he would sit up or walk around to try to find some relief. But deciding what is or is not significant shortness of breath can still be a problem. Again, the physician can help. If the patient is examined during such an episode, a definite decision can usually be made.

The patient's psychological attitude toward his disease

can be the most important problem to be resolved during the convalescent period. Some patients have very definite ideas about their situation that are wrong and dangerous. On one hand is the younger person, usually in his fifties, who will not admit that he has a heart problem. His mind has been grappling with the reality of middle age for some time before his infarction, and this incursion on his health only makes things worse. So his solution is just to reject the whole idea. This is dangerous, because this person is not motivated to do the things that are necessary to improve his chances of avoiding further trouble. Patience and understanding on the part of the family and the doctor may help him realize his problem, but frequently only further illness will drive the message home.

At the other extreme is the person who equates a heart attack with a terrible brush with death and the certainty of impending doom. This person frequently becomes very selfish in his behavior and overprotects himself. He may be perfectly capable of returning to his former work, but he refuses to go back to that job, or frequently, any job. He is not going to take the risk of work causing another coronary! The person may be less aggressive and revert to childlike dependence on his family. This behavior is not based on the facts of what the future may actually be but on preconceived notions. A person such as this may behave this way because of subconscious motivation. In this case, time, reassurance, and persuasion may eventually lead him back to a productive life.

On the other hand, some individuals have long been looking for just such an excuse to avoid the responsibilities of life. When they find that they have survived their myocardial infarct, they are twice relieved, first, because of their recovery, and second, because at last they have their "out" and can retire. This discussion is not intended to condemn such individuals, but to help them, their family, and associates to understand what may be motivating this behavior pattern.

Let us now examine the stark statistics. A certain percentage of persons who have a myocardial infarct will not survive. This number is decreasing, but in general, the mortality rate may be 20 percent with an initial attack. Another 10 to 20 percent of patients will have problems with angina pectoris or heart failure after their infarct. These people will have to restrict their activities to a greater or lesser degree, and medical help can usually increase each individual's capacity. Finally, well over two-thirds of the persons who have experienced a myocardial infarct will be able to return to a near normal life. This is by no means a grim prospect.

Now, a really encouraging thought has evolved over just the past few years. Most people who do not have significant angina or heart failure can improve their health sufficiently to be able to live normal lives! This "normal life" will not be presented to the patient on a silver platter but must be attained by work. All aggravating factors that have been encountered in each individual case must be controlled. This may include weight reduction and maintaining the new weight, abstinence from cigarette smoking, a special diet, a change of pace, taking drugs to control high blood pressure, and most important, physical exercise.

Many persons who have myocardial infarcts are in very poor physical condition. They take no form of exercise other than the amount of walking necessary to do their day-to-day activity. The heart of an athlete is much stronger than that of a desk clerk and will do much more work on demand. After a myocardial infarct, even though part of the heart muscle is damaged and dies, the remaining heart muscle can frequently be trained to overcome the loss, and the person's heart may become stronger than it was before the infarct. In addition, physical exercise tends to decrease body fats and cholesterol and increase a general feeling of well being. Physically active people have less chance of having a myocardial infarct, and if they do have one, a better chance of surviving it.

Physical exercise must be undertaken gradually after a myocardial infarct under the direction of the patient's physician. In some parts of the country, physical rehabilitation centers for cardiac patients have been set up. Exact tests are performed on the patient before the exercise program begins. An estimate is made of his physical capabilities, and then a special gymnasium exercise program is prescribed for him. Tests are made continually to determine whether further increases in activity are warranted or if a plateau should be established. This sort of program will undoubtedly become more widespread in the United States, but meanwhile, the patient's private physician can do a fine job in prescribing increases in exercise.

Sex After Your Coronary

Despite many surveys that have been performed in the past few years, and several books that have been written on the subject of sex, we still lack adequate hard facts regarding the sexual habits of most Americans. If the 1970 census had included questions on the sexual habits of the public, we would know a great deal more than we do. However, the census was never intended to provide this kind of information. The point is, it would take a study of some magnitude to get close to the truth.

We do know that people in their seventies and eighties have sexual intercourse, and certainly people in the twenty- to sixty-year age group do. Since heart attacks develop in persons in the twenty- to eighty-year age group, the consideration of this topic is pertinent to our general discussion.

Some persons will have a decreased desire for sexual intercourse after their heart attack, and others will give it up completely because they were about to anyway. One of the general body responses to serious illness of any type is a loss of sexual desire. The body is saving its strength for more life-threatening battles. But a significant number of people have a strong desire to resume sexual relations after a heart attack. What advice can these persons be given?

"How soon can I resume sexual relations, Doctor? Will it be dangerous for me?" The medical profession does not have exact answers for these questions because the problem has not been studied scientifically. Calculated guesses are made, based on a few known facts and the experience of the physician with other patients who have had the same problem.

What do we know about the body's response to sexual intercourse? Masters and Johnson published data that they obtained from persons during intercourse. The blood pressure and the pulse both increased during the final stages of intercourse. The magnitude of increase was variable from person to person. In some cases, the pulse rate increased to 180 beats per minute and the diastolic blood pressure increased an additional 20 to 50 mm of mercury.

Another study was performed recently of persons who had heart disease. Recording electrocardiograms were attached to these subjects, and a constant record of the ECG was obtained for 18 hours at a time. The idea was to see what happened to the ECG during daily activity, including sexual intercourse. Again, it was shown that the heart rate increased considerably, and in some persons frequent extra systoles and bursts of tachycardia occurred. In some persons, signs of a temporary inadequacy of blood flow to the heart was seen.

A third study demonstrates the diverse answers which may be obtained from medical experiments. Dr. Herman K. Hellerstein of the Case Western Reserve University in Cleveland has long been a medical leader in the area of rehabilitation of persons who have suffered and survived heart attacks. In his study, electrocardiograms made with tape recorders worn by patients during 24- and 48-hour periods revealed a more modest heart response to intercourse. The average was only 117 beats per minute, and the range was from 90 to 144 per minute. The highest rates were usually encountered for only brief periods, usually for no more than from 10 to 15 seconds and the energy cost to patients was calculated to be no more than that used in walking up one flight of stairs.

No doubt the age and physical conditioning of the people tested are some reasons for the differences in these findings. Masters and Johnson used younger subjects without health problems. The majority of persons who have heart attacks are in middle age or beyond, and prior to their heart attacks, they have probably developed sexual techniques with their partners which are less vigorous than those seen in younger persons.

This brings up another interesting aspect of sexual relations. Dr. Lenore Zohman of the Montefiore Hospital in New York points out that a clear distinction should be made between marital and extramarital sex in a person who has had a heart attack. Whereas relations between married couples are usually conducted on a low-key scale, the extramarital rendezvous is often conducted in a more charged atmosphere. There is often a combination of fears about discovery, ability to perform, exhibition of manliness and capacity, which may supercharge the atmosphere of the relationship. In these circumstances, the affair would be more stressful, and heart problems could ensue.

We also know that some people have angina pectoris when they have intercourse. This is not surprising, because these persons usually have angina when they exert themselves at any strenuous activity. Fortunately, nitroglycerine usually relieves the discomfort during intercourse, and many doctors will recommend taking a nitroglycerine before intercourse if the patient regularly has angina during the act. The "before" pill will sometimes prevent the episode of angina.

We know that many people can train their bodies after a heart attack so that they are stronger than they were before the attack. This was discussed in the preceding chapter. Factors known to aggravate the basic atherosclerotic process—such as smoking, obesity, and high blood pressure—are eliminated. A graded program of physical activity is instituted. Certainly the person who trains his body this way will be able to have intercourse as successfully as before his heart attack.

The occurrence of angina pectoris does not invariably follow a heart attack. Most patients will not have this problem. However, this is the most distressing symptom that may interfere with sexual intercourse following a heart attack. Persons with angina develop their chest pain when their pulse and blood pressure are raised to a certain level. This "trigger level" varies from one patient to another, but it is usually constant for the individual. In other words, each time a certain person exercises or becomes emotionally excited and raises his pulse and blood pressure to a critical level specific for him, he will experience angina. By physical training, most people can gradually reduce the acceleration of their pulse that occurs with the same quantity of exercise. Therefore, if a person suffers from angina during sexual intercourse, he may be able to overcome this obstacle with time and physical reconditioning. If you have a very strong desire to resume an active sex life, then let this be a stimulus to carry through the general health plan that your doctor outlines for you.

The decision as to exactly when in your recovery phase you can start to have intercourse must rest with your own doctor. Each case will be different and generalities will always be difficult. One advantage exists today over a generation ago, which is that most people are willing to discuss this problem with their doctors. If sexual intercourse is important to you, you should discuss this with your doctor.

Many people who have had a heart attack have frightened themselves away from intercourse following their first trial. Strange symptoms may have developed during the act. The symptom may have been minor chest discomfort, an awareness of a rapid pulse, or slight shortness of breath. The first performance is usually associated with a great deal of anxiety anyway, and with the development of any symptoms, many people would be terrified. Fear, then, may prevent further experimentation. Experimentation is a good term, because undertaking each new activity during convalescence is an experiment to see how the heart is going to react. Just as you report to your physician the effect that walking up your first flight of steps has on your heart, you should tell him if you feel strange in any way during intercourse. There is a good chance that there may be a simple remedy for your problem. The remedy may consist merely of reassurance.

Alcohol may play an important role in the attainment of satisfactory sexual intercourse after a myocardial infarct. Alcohol poses two potential problems, one physical and the other psychological, in the performance of sexual intercourse, whether or not a person has had a heart attack.

Moderate amounts of alcohol will usually relax people. If there is an element of tension present that might hinder successful sexual relations, then alcohol may be beneficial. In most men, however, an excess of alcohol will make it more difficult to achieve an erection and subsequently to complete the act. This is the physical problem. In the post-infarct patient, this may lead to prolonged foreplay and expending a great deal of unnecessary effort attempting completion of intercourse. A brief, enjoyable experience may be turned into an exhausting marathon.

Unsuccessful intercourse frequently causes great anxiety. The next time intercourse is attempted, the person remembers the last attempt and fears failure again. To brace himself for the occasion he frequently again overindulges in alcohol, thinking that this will help him. He does not realize the real reason for his failure. This is the psychological problem that can then lead to greater difficulties.

All patients with heart disease should avoid excessive alcohol consumption. Under the influence of alcohol, many people are tempted to perform feats that they ordinarily would avoid.

If there is any difficulty during intercourse, the matter requires discussion with your doctor. At times male patients will have difficulty attaining or sustaining an erection. In other cases there might be a complete lack of desire. These symptoms could be due to certain medicines which the patient is taking. In many cases, if the physician is aware of the undesirable side effects of the drugs, changes may be possible. The following case demonstrates some of the problems which may arise if either patient or spouse misunderstands the true state of affairs.

Harold was a 48-year-old cabinetmaker. He had been married for three years to his second wife, a woman ten years younger than he, when he had a heart attack while visiting a brother in Virginia. Harold was hospitalized for three weeks, spending one of those weeks in intensive care. On his return to Florida, he developed symptoms of heart failure. Shortness of breath when he walked and a swelling of his ankles finally brought him to a local physician. He was again hospitalized, and after three weeks he was able to return home for further convalesence. During his second hospitalization, Harold had asked his doctor if he would assist him in filing, on the basis of his disability, for social security retirement benefits. The doctor advised Harold that this was premature and that there was a good chance that he might be able to return to some type of work.

Harold was fortunate. He followed his diet and lost twenty extra pounds which he had been carrying around. He took his medication and was gradually able to resume activity. Six weeks after his second hospital discharge, he was back at full time work in his own trade.

The doctor kept close tabs on Harold, checking him frequently for any signs of a return of his heart failure. Three months after the second hospitalization, Harold surprised his doctor when he reported a great deal of anxiety over his impending divorce. Harold was hesitant to discuss the details of the matter, but after persistent probing, he opened up and told his story. His younger wife had been frightened by Harold's two sicknesses and felt certain that he would either die or become an invalid. In either case, she wouldn't have anyone to take care of her. Harold had noticed an increasing coolness between them, and she had finally discussed her fears the day she left him.

Answering direct questions about their sex life, Harold stated that even though he had been given clearance to resume sexual activities, he had tried intercourse only twice since the second hospital stay. Prior to his heart attack, sex had played an important role in their marriage. The doctor arranged for conferences with each of the partners alone and then together. They decided to give the marriage another try, and at this writing, they appear to be getting along well together.

To prevent this type of problem, it is necessary to keep lines of communication open between patient, wife, and doctor. Bring your fears and problems out into the open. There is often an acceptable solution available.

A final question is often asked concerning intercourse after a heart attack: are there any particular sexual techniques that are better than others for the initial trial when sexual relations are resumed? Again, Masters' and Johnson's work indicates that the entire physical and psychological reaction to sexual intercourse, rather than a particular methodology, results in a stimulation of the pulse and increased blood pressure. Most sexual partners have found in their lives together some technique that is more relaxing and less strenuous for one or the other of the partners. Obviously, these techniques should be tried first after a heart attack.

12

Alcohol and Heart Disease

This topic is introduced primarily to clear up several misconceptions that exist in the minds of some people concerning alcohol. The use of alcohol is very widespread in our society, and we are all aware that many people use considerable amounts of it. It is not uncommon for a physician to encounter a patient with a record of myocardial infarction who claims that his previous physician had prescribed daily doses of alcohol in liberal quantities to help prevent further difficulty. This usually turns out to be an exaggeration, as we shall see in a moment.

Drinking alcohol, whether it be scotch, whiskey, gin, beer, or wine, is composed primarily of water, ethyl alcohol, ethers which impart flavor, and fusel oil or chemical contaminents. The ethyl alcohol is the active ingredient as far as the user is concerned. Alcohol is rapidly absorbed from the stomach and intestines, being detected within the body in as little as five minutes after ingestion. The alcohol distributes itself throughout the entire body and is chemically converted to acetaldehyde by the liver. The liver and other body tissues then burn the acetaldehyde with the production of energy and finally the formation of carbon dioxide and water. Alcohol is as readily used as a foodstuff by the body as is sugar, fat, or protein. Herein lies one of the problems of alcohol. It is handled like any other food, and it therefore adds calories to the body. Diet books will vary slightly in listing the caloric content of alcohol, but an ounce of distilled spirits (such as whiskey and rum) will contribute about 100 calories to the diet.

Since many cardiac patients have an underlying problem of excess weight, the quantity of alcohol used daily must be totaled with their food intake to determine the number of calories being consumed daily. A patient who relates how desperately he is cutting his food consumption down to lose weight will say, "I'm eating only 1000 calories a day, doctor, but I still don't lose any weight." Further questioning may then reveal that the person has done nothing to decrease his usual consumption of eight or ten ounces of whiskey a day.

The most serious effect of prolonged use of alcohol is the development of alcoholism. The alcoholic is a person who has become dependent upon alcohol to the extent that it injures his health and interferes with his ability to do his job, perform his usual social functions, and to get along with other people. A person with any form of heart disease frequently has anxieties about his ability to perform his job adequately and to continue to earn a living. This is usually coupled with increased domestic tension due to financial concern, sexual adjustments, and uncertainty about the future. Many people have learned through habits formed long ago to turn to alcohol for solace at such times. Alcohol does not have a stimulating effect on the brain or the personality. The general effect of alcohol is to depress all brain functions. This depression extends to all thought processes and the ability to reason. At sufficiently high levels of intake, alcohol suppresses the brain into unconsciousness. Initially, people may have a slight uplifted feeling from alcohol because of a blocking of higher brain centers that are concerned with anxiety or worry. The absence of worry is then interpreted as a feeling of increased well-being. There is no stimulatory effect of alcohol on the brain, however. The general effect of alcohol is a depression, and if a person is basically depressed by his state of health, the addition of alcohol may lead to moodiness, unusual aggressiveness, or unnecessary agitation.

Another of the direct dangers of alcohol in persons with heart disease is that some of these persons have definite physical limitations. They may develop angina or symptoms of heart failure if they overexert themselves. Most patients have learned the meaning of their symptoms and regulate their activities so that they do not push themselves too far. Under the influence of alcohol, their judgment may be impaired, and they may not realize that they should not be undertaking a particular activity until it is too late.

Recently, a very interesting study was performed by Drs. Gould, Zahir, DeMartino, and Gomprecht in Bronx, New York. Patients with various types of heart disease and a group of normal people were each given two ounces of whiskey. All the subjects were extensively studied in the cardiac laboratory, and it was found that the whiskey increased the amount of blood pumped by normal hearts, but decreased the heart output in the patients with heart disease.

There is no medically proven beneficial effect of alcohol on the heart. Alcohol does not "open up" the coronary arteries, nor does it have any magical tonic effect. Alcohol makes the arteries in the skin dilate and carry more blood, with the effect that a person who is drinking may feel or look flushed and even perspire more. This does not happen in the heart. Alcohol does act somewhat like a tranquilizer in that it is a general depressant. Anxious people might therefore feel more relaxed, and if anxiety were triggering angina pectoris, such persons could experience less angina if they were properly dosed with alcohol. Moderate amounts of alcohol might be prescribed to a cardiac patient for this reason, but the total effect on the body would have to be evaluated. If the cardiac patient has a problem due to the heart not pumping adequate amounts of blood, then even small amounts of alcohol may very well further aggravate the situation.

It must be remembered also that certain people develop liver damage and brain damage from prolonged use of alcohol, and it is impossible to predict in advance who will be affected in these ways.

Recent scientific studies have demonstrated a type of heart disease that may be associated with the heavy use of alcohol. The studies so far tend to implicate beer as the culprit, used in large quantities. Only certain persons appear to be susceptible to the disease. The effect upon the heart is the death of the small heart muscle fibers, with the replacement of these fibers by scar tissue. The end effect is a condition termed a "myocarditis," a general inflammatory process involving the heart.

Of course, all persons who are in the habit of drinking large quantities of alcohol, even on a daily basis, do not become alcoholics. Each of us probably knows one or two individuals who are able to drink as much as a pint a day and who still function very adequately at their jobs. These people may even be able to consume large amounts of alcohol without any outward appearance of drunkenness. This is probably because they have a body chemistry that burns up alcohol faster, or because their nervous systems have adjusted to function normally despite the presence of alcohol. These people are probably not immune to the alcohol withdrawal syndromes, however.

The alcohol withdrawal syndromes are a final category of problems that confronts the cardiac patient who uses alcohol freely and daily. In an unpredictable fashion, such persons develop withdrawal symptoms when they stop drinking. The symptoms may be mild and consist primarily of tremulousness, or they may appear in the form of nausea and vomiting for several days after alcohol intake has ceased. When withdrawal symptoms are more severe, a state of delerium tremens (D.T.) develops. This is a grave situation characterized by confusion, restlessness, agitation, hallucinations, tremor, sleeplessness, and even convulsions, most often starting three to four days after the person has stopped drinking and lasting another two or three days. The situation appears to be more likely to occur after the person has gone through some stress, such as an operation or a heart attack. The development of delerium tremens in a person who has sustained a heart attack two or three days before is very serious. The agitation and delerium severely tax the heart, and survival from this combination of events occurs but is unusual.

In summary, then, the moderate use of alcohol after a heart attack may not be associated with any significant problem. Physicians may even prescribe alcohol for its tranquilizing effects. As with other drugs, however, an overdose of alcohol may be associated with a variety of difficulties, the least of which is the caloric intake.

13
Atherosclerosis
Outside the Heart

In an earlier chapter we described the disease atherosclerosis, or hardening of the arteries. This is the process by which deposits form on the inside of arteries, resulting in their narrowing down. The development of atherosclerosis in the coronary arteries was seen to be the cause for most myocardial infarctions, or heart attacks. This disease process can affect arteries in other parts of the body, and persons who have had heart attacks frequently have problems with other arteries. Such problems, in fact, may be of greater consequence than the heart disease and will therefore be discussed in detail.

Atherosclerosis can involve any artery in the body. If the arteries supplying the brain with blood are affected, part of the brain may be deprived of adequate blood, and a stroke may result. The artery that feeds the eye with blood may be stricken, in which case sudden blindness may occur. The arteries that nourish the kidneys may be affected. In this instance the disease is usually not symmetrical; in other words, one kidney is affected more than the other. The result of decreased blood flow to a kidney may initially be high blood pressure (hypertension), and eventually that kidney may cease to function altogether.

The liver is seldom affected by atherosclerosis, because it has a double blood supply. Most of the blood that reaches the liver arrives there from the portal vein, and the veins usually do not develop atherosclerosis.

The small intestine is the organ system responsible for digesting our food. Its blood supply comes from the superior and inferior mesenteric arteries that lead off the large aorta in the abdomen. Some unfortunate people develop narrowing of these mesenteric arteries to the extent that the intestine does not receive as much blood as it needs. The inadequate blood supply becomes symptomatic during the process of food digestion, that is, for an hour or two after a person eats. This condition usually produces symptoms that have been given the descriptive name of "abdominal angina." The person typically develops mid-abdominal cramps or pain after eating. The pain is usually not relieved by moving about or by taking antacids or laxatives. It tends the progress rather rapidly and in time may become constant. Since eating induces the pain, persons affected frequently reduce their food intake and lose weight. Food may also be improperly digested and absorbed, and this adds to the weight loss.

When abdominal angina is suspected, the patient is examined by means of an arteriogram. A catheter (small tube) is inserted into the interior of an artery in the groin. The catheter is advanced into the aorta to the point where the mesenteric arteries originate. Dye is then injected rapidly into the catheter and at the same time multiple x-rays are taken. If a narrowed area is found in one of the mesenteric arteries, then surgery is performed on the patient, and the artery is repaired. The same general techniques of artery repair that were previously described for the coronary arteries are used here.

The most common location for atherosclerosis, other than in the heart, is in the arteries that feed the legs. Blood leaving the heart flows into the large aorta, which carries blood to all parts of the body. As the aorta passes down into the abdomen, it divides into two large iliac arteries that supply the pelvis and the legs. When the iliac arteries enter the thighs, their name changes to femoral arteries. The femoral arteries then branch into smaller and smaller vessels that eventually supply the feet and toes. Any of these blood vessels can be affected by atherosclerosis, from the largest (the aorta) to the smallest arteries in the feet.

Arteriosclerosis obliterans is the medical name applied to inadequate blood supply to the legs. The process can also occur in the arms, but does so infrequently. The main symptom that develops in the legs is pain, particularly in the calves, when the person is walking or running. The reason for this is simple. When a person walks or runs, the muscles of his legs are exercising and require more blood flow to supply food and oxygen to the muscles. The heart beats faster and more blood is pumped through the arteries. Just as the heart produces the pain of angina pectoris if it does not get an adequate blood supply during exercise, the leg muscles cause pain if they are getting insufficient blood supply. When the disease process becomes more advanced, the pain in the legs may become constant, occurring even at rest. At this stage, walking is practically impossible.

Another symptom that may be noticed is coldness of the legs and feet, or pain in the legs and feet when they are exposed to cold. For this reason, the afflicted person may keep his feet covered with extra stockings. Feet may appear very red, or even bluish, when the person is standing or sitting. Hair on the feet and toes may disappear and growth of the toenails may be retarded.

A mistake is commonly made at this point. Feeling cold in the feet and legs, people frequently wrap their legs with hot water bottles, hot towels or heating pads, and because the skin and other tissues are easily damaged by outside heat, it is very easy to "cook" the tissue.

The subject of damaged tissue introduces another problem: people with an inadequate blood supply to some part of the body do not heal there as fast as normal because the process of healing requires blood flow. Extra care is therefore necessary to avoid wounding these tissues and to prevent infection.

A stratagem can be followed that will assist healing. The blood flow to the leg is greater when a person is lying down or sitting with his legs up than when he is on his feet or sitting in the usual manner because gravity tends to hold the blood down in the leg and resists its return to the heart. When a person is walking, the muscles of the legs help to pump the blood back to the heart. The veins of the legs have special one-way valves inside of them to facilitate this pumping action. When the leg is elevated, the total blood flow to the leg is increased. Therefore, the person with a cut or infection in a leg with a diminished blood flow due to arteriosclerosis should elevate the damaged limb as often as possible during the day to increase the flow of blood and hasten healing.

If the larger blood vessels (iliac arteries) in the pelvis are affected by atherosclerosis, the person will frequently notice that the pain that he feels when he walks is located in the thighs rather than in the calves. For men, another frequent symptom of blockage in this location is the loss of the ability to have an erection. The process of erection is dependent upon an increased flow of blood into the penis. The artery that supplies this blood is a branch of the iliac vessels.

The ultimate problem that can occur with this condition in the legs is the development of gangrene. This death of tissue caused by inadequate blood flow results in part of the toe or the entire leg turning black. The process usually starts in the toes, and it is frequently immediately preceded by an infection or injury of the tissue in the area. If the blockage is extensive, the gangrene may progress to involve the entire foot or part of the leg. When the disease has progressed to this point, amputation is the only recourse.

The treatment of atherosclerosis of the legs is based first on establishing the diagnosis. A person may consult his doctor because of a condition known as intermittent claudication: at rest his legs feel normal, but when he begins to walk, the calves of his legs develop pain and weakness that is intensified as he continues walking until the pain or weakness forces him to stop. With rest, the pain and weakness disappear from his legs. A second common complaint that might cause a person to go to a doctor is poor healing of a wound or infection on the foot or leg. Many cases are discovered during routine physical examination. The normal pulsation of arteries in the ankle and foot is easily felt by a physician (or by the patient, if he knows where to look). If the pulsating is normal, disease is seldom present, although on occasion it may be necessary to exercise the legs and after the exercise again examine the arteries to find that blood flow is decreased. Instruments are also available that will detect the quantity of blood flow to a limb, and temperature measurements can be made that help in the diagnosis.

The next step is to determine whether or not any conditions exist in the patient that may be aggravating the development of atherosclerosis. Persons with diabetes mellitus have a much higher incidence of atherosclerosis, particularly the type that affects the legs. An elevation of cholesterol level and other body fats in the bloodstream will accentuate the disease, and these should be controlled if possible. Cigarette smoking is another culprit, and this factor can be eliminated. In general, the same factors that aggravate atherosclerosis of the coronary arteries are searched for and eliminated as much as possible. In some patients exercise proves helpful over a period of time. The person walks to the point of leg pain, rests, and then walks again. Over several months, many people find that they are able to walk farther and farther without the development of leg pain, and pulses may even return in their feet.

Despite these measures, in certain individuals the disease progresses and a variable degree of incapacitation develops. These patients are then considered for surgery. Arteriograms are performed to determine the exact areas of the arteries that are narrowed. If the disease affects primarily the larger arteries, or if there is only a short segment of artery that is diseased, a direct approach can be taken. The artery is opened and the obstructing material is removed, or an entire segment of artery may be replaced with a vein or a tube of synthetic material. In some cases, bypasses are established. A vein that is not essential is removed from the opposite leg. One end of the vein is attached above the area of obstruction, and the other end is attached to the diseased artery below the area of obstruction. Blood is now able to shunt around the blocked area. If the disease process is very widespread, however, it may be impossible to operate on enough of the arterial tree to effectively increase circulation in the feet. In these patients, sympathectomy is sometimes of benefit.

The sympathetic nerves are an accessory nervous system that helps regulate blood flow to different parts of the body. The system sends small nerves to the individual branches of the arterial tree. If a person is cold, for example, and it is necessary for the body to conserve heat, these nerves signal the arteries to narrow themselves so that blood flow is decreased to the skin and muscles. Heat is thus conserved. If it is necessary for the person to perspire to lose excess heat, the same nerves will signal the arteries to dilate and allow an increased amount of blood to flow to the skin and sweat glands.

Some patients with atherosclerosis in the arteries of their legs have an abnormal amount of sympathetic nerve stimulation present, and if this stimulation is removed, the arteries will dilate to a certain degree and blood flow in the leg will increase. When a sympathectomy is performed, the nerve pathways are cut to interfere permanently with the transmission of signals to the legs. As indicated above, in a certain percentage of patients this will be beneficial.

Aneurysms. An aneurysm is a local dilatation of an artery or a vein. The reason for the development of an aneurysm is a weakness in the wall of the blood vessel. This could occur, for example, in a knife wound that slices the outside layer of a vessel without cutting all the way through. In time, the pressure inside the vessel causes a bulge in the weakened area. A ballooning effect occurs, and the wall of the vessel progressively thins in the area where the bulge is occurring.

The body tries to compensate for this weakness by forming a scar around the bulge, but eventually a leak or blowout occurs.

Some aneurysms are congenital in origin. In other words, the vessel was improperly formed at birth. The most common location for a congenital aneurysm is in the blood vessels that supply the brain. This type is called a berry aneurysm. Usually occurring in the base of the brain at the bottom of the skull, it is a common cause of strokes in young people. The aneurysm occasionally leaks before it finally blows out, with the development of a severe headache in a person who was previously well and healthy. The usual story is the development of a severe headache followed by unconsciousness, or just sudden unconsciousness in a person in the twenty to forty age group. The person may die within minutes, or regain consciousness, have amnesia, and complain of a headache and stiff neck. The patient may also have transient paralysis of an arm or leg.

The diagnosis of this problem is suspected by the history of events. An aneurysm becomes very suspect if a spinal tap is performed and blood is found in the normally clear fluid that surrounds the brain and spinal cord. In this event, an arteriogram of the blood vessels that supply the brain is undertaken. This will usually show the aneurysm, and then a surgical attack to the problem can be made.

A more common type of aneurysm occurs in some persons who have angina or heart attacks. This is the aortic aneurysm usually caused by atherosclerosis. As we mentioned earlier, when atherosclerotic plaques form inside the arteries, the patches of cholesterol, calcium, and scar tissue protrude not only into the lumen (passageway) of the artery, but also into the wall of the blood vessel. This may produce a weakening of the wall of the vessel. Depending upon the amount of blood pressure that the vessel is exposed to and the extent of wall damage by the patch of atherosclerosis, a ballooning may develop. This most commonly occurs in the aorta as it passes through the abdomen. The aorta, we will recall, is the large blood vessel that carries blood from the heart to all parts of the body via its branches. It passes through the chest, runs down the back of the abdominal cavity, and ends in the iliac arteries that go to the legs. Atherosclerotic aneurysms of the aorta most commonly occur in the abdomen, but may also occur in the chest.

The aneurysm may produce no symptoms, or a person may become aware of a pulsating mass in the abdomen. This recognition is more apt to occur in thin persons. The awareness of the pulsation may be greater when a belt or tight garments are worn. If the aneurysm is rapidly expanding or if it is leaking blood, the patient may experience pain in the abdomen or back. The pain can vary from a mild ache, to a burning or cutting sensation, to a severe pain. The pain is sometimes felt in the back if the leak is occurring through the back of the vessel, where pressure will irritate nerves coming from the nearby spinal cord. The first sign of trouble could present itself as fainting or the rapid development of shock if the aneurysm suddenly starts to leak large amounts of blood. There is no outward sign of blood loss because all the blood escapes into the abdominal cavity.

All abdominal aneurysms do not leak or rupture. Most physicians have seen patients who have refused to have their aneurysms repaired and who have lived many years afterward. It is usually impossible to predict who will or who will not get into trouble. There is no way to know.

If an aneurysm is suspected in an individual, it is sometimes possible to confirm the diagnosis in a relatively simple manner. The body tries to heal the weakened area of the blood vessel, and sometimes in doing this, a layer of calcium is deposited in the wall of the aorta and the aneurysm. This thin layer of calcium can be seen on a plain x-ray of the abdomen as a fine white line. Therefore, at times, a simple x-ray of the abdomen suffices to establish the diagnosis. In other cases, where doubt exists, an aortogram is performed. Here, dye is injected into the aorta and x-ray films are exposed. The entire aorta is illuminated as a white tube, and the aneurysm is seen as a bulge in the side of the tube.

An operation to repair this fault carries much less risk if the patient is operated upon before the aneurysm has started to leak. If the patient is in good general health, the risk of the operation may be only five percent before a leak, and may rise to over 50 percent after rupture has occurred. The operation involved is the removal of the segment of aorta that contains the aneurysm and replacement of this segment with an artificial blood vessel made of Dacron® or Teflon®.

Another type of aneurysm can occur in the aorta—the dissecting aneurysm. It is most apt to occur in association with hypertension, or high blood pressure, when the middle layer of the aorta develops cysts, or small patch-like areas where elastic fibers have died. This condition is called cystic medial necrosis, and it develops as follows.

The wall of the aorta is composed of three layers, a thin inner lining, a media or middle layer composed mainly of elastic tissue and some muscle, and an outer coat. The aorta, especially near the heart, pulsates with each heartbeat. In other words, it expands and contracts each time a volume of blood is pumped into it. This ability to expand and contract is due mainly to the elastic fiber content of the vessel wall. In high blood pressure, this expansion and contraction effect is exaggerated, and in some persons it leads to a premature wearing out of the elastic fibers. This may progress to the development of islands or pockets of dead elastic fibers, the condition called cystic medial necrosis.

The aorta requires a blood supply to nourish itself. This is provided by small blood vessels that run through its wall. When the small pockets of dead elastic tissue develop in the middle coat of the aorta, bleeding may occur into these pockets. The pockets can then start to join each other, and this, in effect, results in a peeling away of the layers of the aorta. The next event that happens in the development of a dissecting aneurysm is for the pockets of blood to burst through and establish a connection with the interior of the aorta. When this happens, blood under high pressure forces its way into the wall of the blood vessel. The pressure peels apart the layers to a greater and greater extent, leading to the development of a double-barreled tube. Furthermore, the inner passageway, the normal channel for blood flow to the entire body, is narrowed down.

The final outcome of this situation is one of three events. The peeling process, or dissection, may stop of its own accord, or it may result in a rupture of the outer layer of the blood vessel with blood escaping someplace into the body. The third possibility is that the dissection may rupture back through the inner lining of the aorta, so that the blood is allowed to escape back into the interior of the aorta where it belongs.

Since dissecting aneurysms usually start in the chest, near the origin of the aorta, the usual symptom is chest pain. This pain is so similar to that caused by a heart attack, or myocardial infarction, that this possibility must be considered in the differential diagnosis of a heart attack. After a time, the differential usually becomes obvious. For one thing, the pain of the dissection will frequently move down the back, and may even be felt in the abdomen if the blood vessel tear is progressing. Another thing that happens is that side branches arising from the aorta are pinched off to a greater or lesser degree. This results in signs of inadequate blood flow to other organs and, for example, the development of a different blood pressure in the right arm than in the left. The dissecting process can even extend back to the heart. If the coronary arteries are compressed at the point where they arise from the aorta, the situation can even be complicated to produce a myocardial infarct.

Formerly, the treatment for this condition was to repair the tear by immediate surgery. It has recently been determined, however, that results are just as good if the high blood pressure that caused the dissection is controlled and surgery not performed. Individual problems will dictate which course of treatment must be followed.

Embolism. An embolus is a clot or other plug brought by the circulation from a distant point and forced into a smaller vessel so as to obstruct circulation in it. The commonest materials that form an embolus in the circulatory system are blood clots and patches of atherosclerosis. If a blood clot is formed any place *within* the heart or blood vessels, a piece may break free and be carried along with the circulation, eventually blocking a smaller vessel. Because we often see people who are afraid that they may develop an embolus from a bruised area, it should be noted that such is not possible. If a person is injured and develops a bluish bruise, even if there is a lump associated with it, this is usually due to trauma breaking a blood vessel, most often a capillary or a small vein. The blood leaks out of the broken vessel into the surrounding tissues and finally clots. The blood clot in the tissue cannot travel to another part of the body, as it would if it were inside the blood vessel, and there is no danger of an embolism. The small injured blood vessel will also develop a clot at the point where the blood escaped, but this is usually tightly adherent to the vessel and will not break loose.

To understand where an embolus will finally lodge, we must understand the difference between veins and arteries. Blood is pumped from the heart to the body. This blood is carried by arteries. In every organ and tissue of the body, the arteries branch into smaller and smaller size vessels, the smallest being the capillaries which are so small that just one blood cell at a time can pass through. The blood is then sent back to the heart, traveling through the veins. The veins get larger as they progress toward the heart. The blood then enters the right side of the heart and is pumped to the lungs. The vessels that supply the lungs break down into smaller and smaller channels until capillaries are again formed. At the level of the capillaries, gas exchange occurs between the blood and the air spaces in the lungs.

If a blood clot occurs in a vein in the leg (thrombophlebitis, or phlebitis) and then breaks loose, this clot, or embolus, will lodge in the lungs. The reason for this is that the clot will be traveling inside of vessels that are larger than the one in which it formed until the lungs are reached; at which point the vessels narrow down to capillary size. Therefore, all clots that form in veins and travel as emboli will lodge in the lungs. An embolus that starts in the heart, however, could end up in any organ in the body, because blood from the heart is pumped to every organ in the body. We will draw the line a little finer now by saying that if a blood clot was formed in the right side of the heart, it would lodge as an embolus in the lungs. If a blood clot originated in the left side of the heart, it would lodge in any organ or part of the body.

Blood clots in veins are discussed in the next chapter. Blood clots form inside the heart and arteries under the following circumstances. One of the body's healing responses with aneurysms is sometimes the formation of blood clots on the interior surface of the aneurysm. If a piece of this clot is released into the circulation from an abdominal aortic aneurysm, the embolus would probably finally lodge in the legs. During a heart attack, sometimes a blood clot is formed on the inside of the heart over the area of muscle that has died. A blood clot in this location is called a mural thrombus. If the heart attack involved the right side of the heart, an embolus from the clot would lodge in the lungs. If the left side of the heart were involved (as it more frequently is), then an embolus from this mural thrombus would pass out to any organ or part of the body. We saw in an earlier chapter how clots sometimes form in the auricles of the right or left atria during atrial fibrillation. An escape of a fragment would go either to the lungs or to the general body, depending on whether it originated in the right or the left atrium.

Approximately 20 percent of persons who suffer a stroke have first had a recent heart attack which may have gone unrecognized. This happens because a person with a heart attack has a 20 percent chance that he will have few symptoms associated with it. These are the silent coronaries that we spoke of earlier. A mural thrombus could form inside his heart over the area of dead muscle, and then a piece of this clot could break off, travel to the brain, and plug up an artery. This would produce death of some brain tissue, and a stroke would result. The first symptoms that might bring a person to a doctor could therefore be paralysis of an arm and leg or unconsciousness. If the stroke affected the area of the brain that controlled the patient's speech, he might not be able to tell the doctor that he had had chest pain two hours before he collapsed with a paralyzed arm and leg.

Atherosclerosis is not a uniform process. It usually occurs in scattered areas with skips between larger and smaller patches of atheroma. The atheromas, plaques of atherosclerosis, usually become hard and brittle as calcium is deposited in the patches of cholesterol. This is in contrast to the normal elasticity of arteries. People can sometimes feel arteries pulsating in neck, shoulders, or arms. This ability to pulsate is due to the elasticity of the vessel. Pieces of an atheroma may break loose from the wall of an artery spontaneously, as a result of the constant pulsation of the vessel, or possibly after an injury, such as a blow over the artery. These pieces now become emboli, and depending upon where they lodge, they may cause a myocardial infarct, a stroke, an infarct in a kidney or the eye, or an embolus to the leg.

An embolus to a leg produces a dramatic sequence of events, resembling the symptoms of arteriosclerosis obliterans but taking place more suddenly. As the particle lodges in an artery in the thigh or calf, it is typically several minutes before anything unusual is noticed. The first indication of trouble is usually a numbness of the leg and foot, a feeling as if it had "gone to sleep." The symptoms commonly occur several inches below the point where the embolus had lodged, due to collateral or accessory blood supply. When the person attempts to walk, the exercise of the leg muscles produces a dull aching sensation and finally a definite pain in the lower leg. This pain is initially relieved by resting, but then it becomes more constant, and the leg may feel too weak to support body weight. Within a matter of a few hours, the temperature of the affected leg is noted to be cooler to the touch of the hand than the normal leg. The skin color may become slightly bluish, or if the leg is hanging down, it may be a red-blue color. People are frequently tempted to apply heat to the affected leg to "improve the circulation," but we have seen that this may hasten tissue injury.

The diagnosis is usually readily apparent to the physician because of the localized symptoms the difference in the temperature and appearance of the affected leg, and the (usual) lack of pulses in the lower leg. The treatment of the condition is, first, rest and protection of the leg. Anticoagulants (drugs that delay blood clotting) are frequently prescribed because blood has a tendency to clot in the artery above and below the point where the embolus lodged. Arteriograms determine the exact site of the embolus and make it possible to evaluate the other arteries in the leg. The problem at times resolves itself, possibly because the embolus fragments and the smaller particles filter lower down in the circulation of the leg to plug less critical small arteries and capillaries. At other times, surgery is necessary to attempt to remove the embolus and any secondary clots that have formed.

14
Pulmonary Embolisms—
Pulmonary Infarcts

Pulmonary embolisms are blood clots that lodge in the lungs. The clots originate in one of the veins of the body or in the right side of the heart. Sometimes the embolism in the lung causes death of a segment of lung tissue, in which case a pulmonary infarct has occurred. A few examples will demonstrate the diverse circumstances in which pulmonary emboli can occur.

Keith M., a 60-year-old man, was in the hospital convalescing from a myocardial infarct. He had entered the hospital two weeks before complaining of a squeezing pain across the front of his chest that had persisted for three hours. He had never before experienced this sensation, and he had fainted twice at home before he summoned help to transport him to the hospital. He had been admitted to the hospital's coronary care unit, and after initial medication for pain, had been comfortable. He was moved into a regular hospital room on the seventh day after his heart attack. Now he was allowed to go to the bathroom and to sit in a chair during his meals.

Keith had just returned to his bed after lunch, when he suddenly felt a severe pain developing in the right side of his chest. The pain did not go away, and whenever he tried to take a deep breath, the pain was aggravated. He felt slightly short of breath and rang the bell for the nurse. After he had explained his symptoms, the nurse connected an oxygen tube to his nostrils and checked his pulse and blood pressure. His blood pressure was satisfactory, but his pulse had increased to 120 beats per minute. Since his transfer to this room, his pulse rate had usually been in the 80 to 90 range. The nurse also noted that his respiration rate had increased. The patient's doctor was summoned and an injection of a pain-relieving drug was administered.

Keith's doctor arrived in a short time and examined him. He thought he knew what the problem was and that it could be taken care of. Later that afternoon, Keith began to cough up sputum that had traces of red blood in it. Blood tests were taken, as well as an electrocardiogram. A small x-ray machine was brought up to his hospital room and a picture was taken without moving him from his bed. Later that day his doctor returned and told Keith that a small blood clot had traveled to his lung and had lodged there, and that these symptoms were the result. The blood clot would probably disappear in time, and he would be given special medicine (anticoagulants) to prevent any further blood clots from forming.

Keith was uncomfortable for three days, but the symptoms gradually subsided and he had no further difficulties before his discharge. His doctor was not sure where the blood clot had originated, but because of the strong possibility that it had arisen in the veins of his legs, he was given elastic stockings to wear. The stockings were a nuisance, but Keith soon adapted to them, and wore them all the time except when he bathed himself.

Sylvia M., 32, had delivered her third child, a boy, four weeks ago. There were no problems associated with the delivery, and she took her son home with her on the fourth day after his birth. She soon began to notice a pain in her back, just below the shoulder blades, and thought that it was just a backache caused by lifting the baby. After two days the pain disappeared. The following week, she developed a slight cough and began to experience chilliness in the afternoons. Several days later she had a catching pain in her left side and started to cough up clear mucous that occasionally had particles of blood in it. The same day that the blood appeared in her sputum, she felt unusually hot in the afternoon, and when she took her temperature, she found that it was 102 degrees.

Sylvia called her doctor, who advised her to see him the same day. At his office, the doctor took a chest x-ray and told her that she should go back to the hospital. The x-ray had shown a shadow in her left lung, and the doctor thought that she had a pulmonary infarct. Sylvia's course in the hospital was very smooth, and she was able to return home a week later.

Joan W. came to the hospital emergency room late one night. She reported that she had developed chills and fever three days earlier and that the fever seemed to subside each time she took aspirin. The following day she developed a pain in the right side of her chest that appeared to be worse when she took a deep breath. She also felt that she was more short of breath than she should be. Joan had decided to come to the emergency room that night because she was more uncomfortable and was starting to cough up brown and red sputum.

After the emergency room doctor had examined her chest, he had an x-ray taken and reported that he thought she had a pneumonia. She was admitted to the hospital.

Later that evening Dr. Brown came into her room, introduced himself, and began to review her symptoms with her. As the interview proceeded, Joan reluctantly revealed that she also had a vaginal discharge that had been present for three days. Dr. Brown asked her about her menstrual periods, and finally Joan disclosed that four days earlier she had had an abortion performed. She was married and had three children, and amazingly, this was her fourth abortion. She felt well enough the day of the abortion to return home but now expressed the fear that things may not have gone as well as on previous occasions. After Dr. Brown had performed a pelvic examination that was rather painful, he told Joan that she had an infection in her uterus, and that he was afraid it had spread into the veins in her pelvis. Her lung problem was probably not a pneumonia, but rather, infected blood clots that had lodged in her lungs.

Dr. Brown's diagnosis proved to be correct. Joan was treated with antibiotics and anticoagulants, and eventually she recovered. However, she was hospitalized for five weeks because the infected blood clots had formed multiple abscesses in her lungs, and they took a long time to respond to treatment.

Pulmonary embolisms and pulmonary infarcts are commonly encountered problems in hospitals. They are prone to occur in any person who is bedridden for a week or more.

The incidence is probably highest in persons with heart failure because the circulation in heart failure is sluggish. In this situation, there is a back pressure in the veins that drain into the heart, and it takes longer for blood to complete a normal circuit from the left side of the heart to the body and back to the heart again via the veins. People with heart failure also spend most of the day either lying in bed or sitting in a chair. The blood tends to pool in the legs in this circumstance. Normally, when a person is up and walking about, the muscles in the legs contract and tend to force blood back up to the heart. Slowed circulation and inactivity predispose the patient to development of blood clots in the deep veins of the legs.

Blood clots in the leg veins, thrombophlebitis, may occur without any symptom or indication in the leg that anything is wrong. On the other hand, the involved leg may become painful, especially on walking. In addition, the lower leg may swell, and the leg may feel warmer. At times, a redness of the lower leg may be seen. The calf is frequently tender, but not necessarily so. One of the indications that a vein may be clotted or otherwise inflamed is the occurrence of "Homan's sign" in the involved leg. This physical test is performed by extending the leg straight out while the person is lying on his back. The end of the foot and the toes are then bent up by the patient towards his head. A pain in the calf or behind the knee indicate a positive Homan's sign.

Many readers will recall that it used to be common practice to keep women who had recently delivered babies, and patients who had recently undergone surgery, in bed for several weeks after the event. Pulmonary embolisms and pulmonary infarcts were more common in those days. When it was realized the part that inactivity played in the development of this process, early ambulation was started. This simple step, getting people out of bed as soon as possible, sharply reduced the incidence of blood clot problems. The situation is still with us, however. In autopsy studies of large numbers of persons who have died from various causes, it is common to find pulmonary emboli in the lungs of up to 50 percent of these people. Blood clots in the lungs were the cause of death in 10 to 15 percent of these persons.

The case histories of Sylvia and Joan demonstrate that blood clots can develop in the pelvic veins. During pregnancy the uterus enlarges greatly, even during the early months, and the blood supply to it is greatly increased. When the uterus is emptied, either spontaneously by delivery or artificially by abortion, the uterus rapidly decreases in size, but days are required for the organ and its blood vessels to reduce themselves to normal size. During this period, pooling of blood can occur in the veins, and under certain situations, blood clots may form. If the uterus becomes infected for any reason, it is very easy for the infection to extend into the blood vessels associated with the uterus. This is not a common complication of normal deliveries, but it does occur. If a blood clot in the pelvis or any other part of the body is infected, and if part of this clot breaks loose and travels to the lungs, the infection is carried with it. The area of lung involved then usually becomes infected with the same organism that was causing the pelvic infection. The lung condition in some ways resembles a pneumonia, but there is the associated obstruction of a blood vessel.

In order to keep this problem in proper perspective, it is important to point out that most persons have many pulmonary embolisms during their lifetime that they are unaware of. It is a common occurrence. Each of us may have from 10 to 50 of these blood clots lodge in our lungs and never realize that anything has happened. On the other hand, we may be aware of a fleeting chest pain of several minutes duration that then disappears, and we forget about the entire matter. I can recall several instances when I am sure that I had a small embolus strike my lungs. It usually occurred during an automobile trip. While driving, I would suddenly get a pain someplace in my chest that was sharp and stabbing, and then within minutes it would be gone. These clots were probably very small, and they may very well have fragmented and disappeared after sticking in a small blood vessel in the lung.

If a pulmonary embolism occurs in persons who are otherwise healthy, it is common for it to develop in relation to some circumstance that involves unusual inactivity. This may be an extended trip by car, plane, or train, or attendance at a convention or other session where an unusual amount of time is spent seated. In each of these circumstances, the lower legs are vertical and inactive, and blood pools in the leg veins. The obvious preventative measure is to remember to move the feet up and down to pump the blood out of the legs, or to get up and walk around whenever possible.

What effects do pulmonary embolisms have on the heart and the lungs? A small embolus causes minimal problems, while a large embolus may cause death. The immediate problem is the obstruction of a blood vessel. Blood will no longer flow into a segment of lung tissue. Air will still pass in and out of this portion of the lung, but oxygen will not be extracted from the small air pockets. This is because the oxygen must be picked up by the blood that normally passes through the lung tissue. If a small blood vessel is blocked, the patient may not feel uncomfortable, but if a larger vessel is blocked, he will feel short of breath.

The right side of the heart has the responsibility of pumping blood into the lungs. If a medium size blood vessel is plugged with a clot, or if multiple small arteries are blocked for the same reason, the heart feels a greater resistance working against it as it attempts to empty itself with each contraction. This increased resistance to blood flow puts a strain on the right side of the heart. The heart is able to compensate to a certain extent, but beyond a set point it will weaken. That sequence of events then leads to heart failure with a backup of blood behind the heart. The symptoms of right heart failure from pulmonary embolisms are the same as the symptoms of right heart failure from any cause, namely, edema of the legs and swelling of the liver and abdomen.

The left side of the heart may also be affected by this process. For one thing, if a large clot is present in the lungs, it may so obstruct blood flow through the lungs that the left heart does not receive an adequate blood supply. In other words, there is not enough blood flow to fill the left side of the heart before each contraction. The result of this will be a decrease in the amount of blood pumped by the left side of the heart. This may result in a fall in blood pressure and shock. In extreme circumstances, this could produce unconsciousness, because the brain does not receive enough blood. In addition, this could also produce a heart attack or myocardial infarct, if blood flow in the coronary arteries was diminished excessively. A myocardial infarct would be more likely to occur in a portion of the heart in which the coronary artery branches had already narrowed, resulting in a borderline blood supply to that particular area of the heart.

The next patient's story will illustrate the recurrent nature of pulmonary embolisms, and some interesting facets of its occurrence.

Richard W. was a 40-year-old insurance broker. He and his wife were returning from Europe when he first experienced ill health. On the airplane trip home, he developed a hacking cough and a slight shortness of breath. He passed these symptoms off as minor. The weather in London had been rather miserable, and he had probably picked up a cold. He had been smoking more than usual lately, and that was probably the reason for his shortness of breath. The cough hung on, however, and he developed a catch in his left chest when he coughed or took a deep breath. Four days later he consulted his family doctor after he developed an afternoon fever and chills.

Dr. Burke diagnosed his case as pneumonia. He showed him his chest x-ray, and Richard could see a small dark spot on the film at the bottom of what his doctor said was his left lung. He agreed to stay home the balance of that week and faithfully took his antibiotic capsules and the cough medicine. A week later he was not well, but both he and his doctor felt that progress was satisfactory. After his second week of antibiotics, he was allowed to return to work. His physician said that the lung spot had not cleared up yet and requested that he return in another week to get another chest x-ray. He informed Richard that if the spot did not clear up, something else might be wrong. What could that mean? Cancer?

Luckily, that last x-ray showed that the spot on his lung had disappeared and Dr. Burke finally released him.

About ten days later, his right calf became sore when he was walking. At first, the soreness disappeared when he sat down or stopped walking, but then the pain persisted. He found that if he propped his leg up while he was sitting at his desk, it felt better. That night, he noticed that his right ankle was swollen. Three more days passed and the leg was not getting better, so Richard returned to his doctor. Much to his surprise, Dr. Burke told him that he had a blood clot in the deep veins of his right leg, and that, furthermore, his pneumonia had probably represented a blood clot that had traveled to his lung. The phlebitis had been present in his leg before the lung problem started, but he had been unaware of its presence. Dr. Burke further postulated that the clot may have formed during his vacation in Europe, during which time he had spent a number of days seated in different vehicles.

Richard was hospitalized and treated with anticoagulants. He had to rest and to wear an elastic stocking. Two months after his discharge from the hospital, the anticoagulant drugs were discontinued, and four months later he was able to cast aside the elastic stocking.

Three years later, he had another bout of phlebitis in the right leg. There seemed to be no particular reason for it. This time, his doctor told him just to stay home and rest, but he had to wear the elastic stocking and take the anticoagulants again. In time, he was able again to stop both forms of treatment.

Over the following six years, Richard experienced a gradually increasing shortness of breath. A flight of stairs that previously was easy to climb became a mountain to be gradually ascended. He attributed the problem to his smoking cigarettes and finally he gave them up. After three months, he was disappointed to find that smoking did not seem to make much difference, so he finally followed his wife's advice and went back to Dr. Burke. After an extensive examination, Dr. Burke told him that he was probably developing emphysema and advised him to stay off the tobacco. The doctor added something puzzling, however. He said that maybe he was continuing to have small pulmonary embolisms from his right leg. Richard was surprised to hear that he could have a vein that formed blood clots in his leg without his being aware of any discomfort in the leg. He was further surprised to learn that small blood clots could be striking his lungs without his knowledge or awareness of chest discomfort. Dr. Burke advised that he resume wearing the elastic stocking on his leg, and to report to him any chest pains that he experienced. Richard took his advice for several months, but then he quit the stocking, since it was a bore and a nuisance.

Two more years passed. During this time, Richard had been briefly hospitalized for pneumonia that developed while he was traveling in another part of the country. He had a different doctor and Richard neglected to tell this physician about his previous problems. He just wanted to get better and be on his way.

Finally, luck really failed him, and he was back in the hospital again. This time it was a bad gallbladder, and Richard had to have an operation. The recovery phase was prolonged because of a wound infection. After the third week, the doctors were finally talking about his going home in a few days. That night a horrifying thing happened. Richard was turning over in his bed to go to sleep when he was seized by a severe tightness in the chest, and he became frantically short of breath. He was barely able to signal for the nurse. Fortunately, she answered his summons promptly, and soon his doctors were in attendance.

Richard was not aware of what followed. He lapsed into a state of unconsciousness. The nurses had started oxygen, and after Dr. Burke examined the patient, he began an intravenous solution with medicine added to help support the patient's falling blood pressure. Richard was transferred to the x-ray department where an emergency pulmonary arteriogram was performed. A tube was inserted into a vein and threaded through to the right side of the heart and then past the heart into the lungs. Dye was then injected into the tube and x-rays taken. The films showed that the opaque dye (hence also the blood) had been blocked in a certain area, confirming the diagnosis of a large pulmonary embolism. A special surgical team had previously been alerted and they were ready in the operating room to proceed immediately.

In the operating room, Richard was connected to an artificial heart-lung machine. This machine pumps blood through the body after the blood passes through an artificial lung that extracts carbon dioxide and adds oxygen to the blood. The machine is connected to the patient by tubes that are inserted into large blood vessels. With the patient's chest opened, the large pulmonary artery that leaves the heart and supplies the lungs with blood was identified. This artery was opened after the heart had been artificially stopped. The artery did not leak blood through the opening that the surgeon made, because the heart was not pumping blood. A large blood clot was seen lying in the artery, and the surgeon extracted it, trying to get it out in its entirety. Part of the clot extended back into the right side of the heart, and this portion was removed also. Then with a suction apparatus attached to a tube, the surgeon explored the smaller branches of the pulmonary artery to get out any remaining clots. After he was satisfied that he had removed all the clots, the surgeon closed the incision in the artery with fine sutures. The heart was then restarted, and the team was gratified to see how nicely the heart performed. After waiting several minutes for the body to readjust itself, the artificial heart-lung machine was disconnected and the patient was on his own again.

As the team was closing the chest incision, the surgeon and Dr. Burke discussed what they would do to try to prevent this circumstance from recurring. They would certainly restart Richard on anticoagulants, but would that be adequate to prevent another massive embolus? Both doctors agreed that this might not be sufficient. They decided to put a special device between Richard's right leg, the probable origin of these clots, and his lungs, which had been trapping the freed clots. The device was the recently invented "umbrella screen," which would be inserted into the inferior vena cava. The inferior vena cava is a large vein in the abdomen that receives blood from the legs and abdominal organs and carries it back up to the heart.

The usual method of screening the inferior vena cava was to perform an abdominal operation, identify the vein, and then sew multiple sutures (stitches) in a line across a segment of it. The sutures were pulled tight, but not tight enough to completely block the blood flow. The sutures were supposed to act as a screen and hold any large clots from passing by that point.

By being small enough when folded to be put in place through a neck vein, the umbrella screen makes an abdominal operation unnecessary. No larger than the stub of a pencil, the device is moved into place, then opened like an umbrella. Holes in the umbrella allow blood to flow through but block the passage of clots.

An incision was made in Richard's neck and a large vein was found. A small slit was made in the wall of the vein, and the folded umbrella attached to its special wire was inserted into the vein. The umbrella was advanced down this vein while the surgeon watched its progress through a fluoroscope. The metal device was easily followed on the fluoroscope screen as it passed through the right atrium of the heart and then back out of the atrium through the inferior vena cava that joins the atrium. When the proper position in the inferior vena cava was reached, the umbrella was opened. Around its outer edge were small spikes that caused it to stick into the wall of the vein to hold it permanently in place. The wire was then twisted and unscrewed from the umbrella. The wire was removed, and the small slit in the vein and the neck incision were sewn closed. Richard now had a blocking device to prevent any more large blood clots from reaching his lungs, and his body had been spared the additional affront of an abdominal operation. He fortunately made a fine recovery.

In summary, then, blood clots are apt to develop in the legs of persons who lie in bed for prolonged periods. Such clots are a common complication that occurs in persons who are hospitalized for various reasons. They can also occur in persons who are not hospitalized, but who may be more inactive than usual. Blood clots may also occur in the pelvic veins, especially in women who have just delivered babies, or in women who have infections in their pelvic organs. When a particle of blood clot becomes detached, it is carried up to the lungs, where it lodges. If the embolus is small, nothing serious occurs. If it is large, or if multiple emboli lodge in the lungs, the results can be very serious.

Since many pulmonary embolisms go unrecognized, it is sometimes very difficult to establish this diagnosis. The symptoms often resemble those of pneumonia. Large pulmonary embolisms can produce symptoms very much like those of a heart attack.

One of the reasons why a pulmonary embolism may be hard to diagnose is that the chest x-ray may not show any changes. The x-ray may appear normal if a blood clot lodges in an artery in the lungs and does not cause any damage to lung tissue. If the segment of lung that has its blood flow blocked does not receive adequate nourishment from surrounding blood vessels, then it dies; a pulmonary infarct has occurred. This does produce a change on the chest x-ray. A shadow now appears, but this shadow may be identical to the shadow seen in a lung affected by pneumonia. Furthermore, the symptoms of a pulmonary infarct and pneumonia are very similar. If the patient has indications of a blood clot in some other part of the body, the diagnosis of pulmonary embolism can be deduced. But as we saw above, sometimes this is not obvious. At times, the blood clot from a leg may not reveal itself for days or weeks after it has resulted in a pulmonary embolus.

A final question must be answered on this subject. What are varicose veins, and what part do they play in pulmonary embolism and infarction? Varicose veins are dilated veins that usually develop in the legs. They look like crooked, curled, blue snakes lying beneath the surface of the skin. They are usually soft, and they can be flattened out with pressure applied over them. They are veins that are distended with blood and have become longer than they are supposed to be. The lengthening of the vein produces the corkscrew appearance.

The basic reason for the development of varicose veins is that one-way valves in the veins have been damaged and no longer function. To understand the importance of these valves, we must realize that blood has a long distance to travel when it leaves the feet and starts toward the heart. If the person is standing, and if we remember that gravity is playing a role, it is easy to see that getting this blood up to the heart is a big task. To facilitate this, the leg veins contain valves that allow blood to flow toward the heart but not backward toward the feet. The major veins run deep inside the calves and thighs and are surrounded by muscle. Whenever we walk or otherwise contract the muscles in our legs, these muscles exert pressure on the outside of the veins and actually pump the blood along toward the heart. If the valves are damaged, the veins become distended with blood. This increases the pressure inside the veins and, in time, bulges and stretches them.

Persons born with weak or poorly functioning valves usually develop the varicose veins that we are familiar with when they reach early adulthood. Women with a tendency toward varicose veins frequently notice that the veins are much worse when they are pregnant. This is because the fetus in the enlarged uterus is lying on top of pelvic veins that receive blood from the legs. This pressure slows down the blood flow from the legs and exerts a back pressure that further weakens the valves inside the veins.

Another reason for the development of varicose veins in some persons is the occurrence of blood clots in the major veins in the legs. The presence of blood clots is frequently associated with some degree of inflammation, and this damages the valves in the veins. After an episode of phlebitis, therefore, a person may notice either the development of varicose veins or a swelling of the involved leg. Both symptoms are due to the same factor—increased difficulty with blood flow out of the leg and an increase in pressure in the veins.

Varicose veins on the surface of the legs are seldom a cause of pulmonary embolisms or blood clots. It is true that blood clots may form in a segment of a varicose vein. The patient is usually aware of this phenomenon because he can see and feel a hard area in part of a vein that used to be soft. The area may also be red and warm. This is a blood clot. But, for some reason, these blood clots in superficial varicose veins seldom detach themselves and travel anywhere. They are safe blood clots.

What actually causes the blood clots to form? One factor is certainly a slowing down of the blood flow through the veins. A person lying down in a bed or sitting in a chair has a slower circulation of blood through the legs than a person who is up and walking about. This is because active muscles require more blood flow, and the exercise is constantly pumping the blood out of the legs and back to the heart. Another factor may be some increase in clotting substances in the blood stream. Not much is known about this, but it is known that there is a normal balance in the body between factors that cause blood to clot and factors that normally dissolve clots. In fact, blood clots are being formed in different parts of our body at all times in response to various types of injury. As healing occurs in these areas, substances in the bloodstream dissolve clots that are no longer needed. There may be an imbalance in these factors when clots form in leg veins. This is one reason why anticoagulants (drugs that delay blood clotting) are prescribed for this condition.

The concept that blood flow through veins is slower than

normal when clots form is the reason for using elastic stockings as a method of treatment. The elastic stockings accelerate blood flow in the legs, as has been explained.

When an elastic stocking is worn, all the tissues of the leg are compressed. The veins are all flattened and become narrower. The blood flow through these veins must accelerate, and with this increased speed, blood clotting is less likely to occur. For this reason, doctors will frequently prescribe elastic stockings for persons who are in a situation where they have a greater than normal risk of developing blood clots in the legs and subsequent pulmonary embolisms. Once blood clots have formed, elastic stockings are usually prescribed to prevent their recurrence. The decision as to when a person can discontinue using the elastic stockings is difficult and must be left to the judgment of the physician who prescribed them.

15

Diabetes Mellitus

Diabetes is discussed here for two basic reasons. First, many people with heart attacks have diabetes, and second, the presence of diabetes makes a person more susceptible to a heart attack or any other disease caused by atherosclerosis.

The name diabetes was first applied to the condition by the ancient Greeks. In Greek, this word means "to run through," and Aretaeus about A.D. 70 recognized that persons with this condition appeared to pass larger quantities of urine than normal. In the sixteenth century it was learned that urine of diabetics contained excess amounts of sugar, and the word mellitus, which refers to sweetness, was added to the word diabetes.

It is estimated that about two percent of Americans have diabetes mellitus, and so, with a population of 200,000,000 persons, about 4,000,000 diabetics exist in this country. It is estimated also that about half of this number are not aware that they have the disease.

Atherosclerosis, the disease of arteries that leads to their becoming plugged up and thus causing heart attacks, occurs very frequently in diabetics. This is the problem. A person with diabetes mellitus has a three or four times greater chance of having a heart attack than a person who does not. Furthermore, in diabetics, atherosclerosis occurs at an earlier age, to a greater extent, and to an equal degree in both sexes. In other words, diabetes accelerates the development of atherosclerosis, which occurs in severe form in young persons regardless of sex. Diabetes is thus a great equalizer. Women are ordinarily protected from developing atherosclerosis until after their menopause. They then start to develop the disease, but they do not have as many heart attacks as men do. If a woman has diabetes, however, regardless of her status concerning the menopause, she will have an accelerated rate of development of atherosclerosis and thus heart attacks.

The term "diabetes mellitus" actually covers several different disease processes. In this way it is similar to the term "common cold," which refers to a symptom complex, with a running nose, a feeling of general sickness, perhaps a fever, and usually a cough. We believe that the common cold is due to a virus infection, but actually a number of different viruses have been isolated that will produce the same symptoms. In a similar way, diabetes mellitus means that a person has an excess of sugar in his bloodstream, and that, if the condition is sufficiently advanced, the sugar will appear in his urine. Several different processes will result in these findings. The term thus covers several disease states. The reason for this overlap is that doctors recognized the symptoms before they knew the cause of the disease. Even today, the exact causes of most cases of diabetes mellitus are not known.

In the 1920s Banting, Best, and Macleod were able to prepare a substance, extracted from the pancreas of dogs, that was able to reduce the level of blood sugar in human beings.

That substance was insulin. We do know that most persons with diabetes mellitus will benefit from injections of insulin, but we do not know why their own bodies are not producing an adequate amount of this hormone.

Insulin is produced in the pancreas, a gland located in the abdomen behind the stomach. The insulin is formed in a particular part of the pancreas, and in response to an increased level of sugar in the blood, this hormone is released into the bloodstream. The release of insulin is normally followed by a reduction in the amount of sugar in the blood. The sugar disappears into the liver, the muscles, and the fat deposits of the body.

Some people develop diabetes who have diseases of the pancreas, such as a chronic inflammation of the gland, called chronic pancreatitis, or who have cancer of the pancreas. These patients have a form of diabetes mellitus which is easy to understand. The gland has been destroyed and therefore it cannot produce insulin. They usually have no trouble controlling their sugar problem with injected insulin.

The chemical structure of human insulin was not discovered until 1960. Shortly after that, a method was discovered to measure the amount of human insulin circulating in the bloodstream or present in the pancreas. Prior to this time the disease had been studied by indirect means, but now scientists can measure the deficits or excesses of insulin in diabetics.

In general, two basic forms of diabetes mellitus exist. One form occurs mostly in adolescents, and the second later in life. The first is called juvenile, or growth-onset, diabetes mellitus, and the second form is called maturity-onset, or adult, diabetes mellitus. The difference between these two types is very interesting. The adult form of the disease is usually characterized by a gradual onset, and studies of the blood and pancreas in these persons typically demonstrate the presence of insulin, but in decreased amounts. These findings are compatible with the long-held theory about the origin of diabetes mellitus in that the disease is due to a premature wearing out of the pancreas with its resultant decrease in insulin production.

In the case of juvenile onset diabetes, examiners were surprised to find that some patients with this disease, shortly after its onset, had a normal amount of insulin circulating in their blood and that their pancreas also contained normal, or greater than normal, amounts of insulin. In a period of months, however, insulin completely disappeared from their blood and from their pancreas. This finding led to the postulation that there might be something present in these young people that was using up an abnormal amount of insulin, with the result that the pancreas becomes exhausted from over-stimulation and finally is unable to produce any insulin at all. This unknown agent could be a substance in the body that combines with insulin to prevent it from acting in a normal manner, or perhaps another organ in the body, such as the liver, might remove the insulin from the blood before it has a chance to function.

Another characteristic of this disease is its tendency to occur in relatives of persons who have the disease, or to be inherited. Relatives of diabetics have a chance of developing diabetes two and a half times greater than that of the general population. This inherited disease may first show symptoms at any age. A grandparent may have the disease, and then diabetes may occur in a grandchild during early adolescence. Finally, the child's parent may develop the disease several years after it appeared in the child.

The effect of insulin on various body tissues is interesting. Muscle tissue requires insulin in order to absorb sugar, which it uses as a food and burns to produce energy. Muscles are composed mainly of protein, which is constructed from amino acids. Amino acids may be thought of as building blocks for the production of protein. Muscle tissue apparently requires insulin also in order to use amino acids for the production of more muscle cells. If a person has severe diabetes and is not receiving insulin injections, his muscles will waste away because he is not able to rebuild the tissue, and furthermore, he will experience weakness because his muscles are not able to function properly without adequate food.

The liver ordinarily stores sugar in the form of glycogen. If the blood sugar level falls below normal (as would occur when a person is fasting or if there was an excess production of insulin), then the liver releases sugar into the bloodstream. The source of the sugar is twofold. Glycogen is broken down into glucose (sugar), and the liver is able to convert amino acids (the building blocks for protein) into sugar.

The liver will also release sugar (glucose) in the absence of normal amounts of insulin. Therefore, in the diabetic person, who has inadequate amounts of insulin circulating in his system, the liver will respond by increasing the amount of sugar circulating in the blood. Thus the elevated blood sugar in diabetics is caused by this liver mechanism, and by the tissues, mainly muscle and fat, which do not use up sugar as they normally would if adequate insulin were present.

Although fatty tissue is composed mainly of fat, it also contains a quantity of glucose (sugar). When adequate amounts of insulin are present, sugar is incorporated into the fat deposits of the body. If there is a deficiency of insulin, then sugar cannot be taken up by the fat deposits, and furthermore, the fat deposits break down. Thus, the diabetic loses weight, and he ends up with an excess amount of fat substances circulating in his bloodstream. This may be one reason for the accelerated development of atherosclerosis in the diabetic person. The excess fats may be deposited in the walls of the arteries, forming atheromas, or patches, that constitute the disease of atherosclerosis.

Most persons who develop diabetes mellitus are overweight or have been at some time in their lives. This does not mean that every fat person will develop diabetes. However, if a fat person has a hereditary tendency to ,develop diabetes, the extra weight may cause it to occur sooner.

Two theories attempt to explain the relationship between fat and the development of diabetes. One is that a person who overeats is constantly stimulating his pancreas to produce more and more insulin to take care of the food that is consumed. This tends to wear out the pancreas prematurely. At the same time, however, the insulin that is produced appears to be less effective than it should be, so that more and more insulin is needed to do the same job. Both factors result in a relative deficiency of insulin, with development of the manifestations of diabetes mellitus.

The other theory is that the hereditary factor for diabetes is present in the blood as an anti-insulin factor. This substance will not alter insulin's effectiveness in incorporating sugar into fat, but it will block the action of insulin in muscle tissues. Although insulin is present in the body, it will not induce muscle tissue to take up sugar (glucose). This raises the blood sugar level higher than it should be. The elevated blood sugar then stimulates the pancreas to produce more insulin. The extra insulin pushes the sugar into the fat tissues of the body, leading to weight gain and an increase in the total fat content of the body. In this instance, the diabetic trait is helping to make the person fatter. Eventually, the pancreas fatigues and inadequate amounts of insulin are produced, leading again to the development of overt diabetes mellitus.

Now that we understand something concerning diabetes, how do we discover whether or not we have it? Actually, most people with a diabetic problem are discovered before the disease produces marked symptoms. Doctors in routine examinations of any type check at least the urine for excess sugar, and many times they also do screening tests on the blood to detect diabetes. In particular, if a person goes to a doctor with symptoms suggesting diabetes mellitus, or if he has any symptom that is not easily explained, tests are run to determine whether or not this disease is operative. When persons are admitted to hospitals for any reason, illness or an operation, tests for diabetes are run as a routine part of the admission laboratory work-up.

Should the disease happen not to be picked up in this manner, then the person involved may at first experience only a general feeling of ill health. He does not have the stamina that he used to have. He may have a problem with recurrent infections of any type, especially skin infections, such as boils. Women may encounter repeated bladder infections or vaginal infections. If diabetes is advanced, the urine contains large amounts of sugar, and bacteria grow best in an environment rich in sugar. This is the reason for the infection problem.

When the disease is advanced, the classical symptoms of diabetes appear. The person is very thirsty, drinking unusual quantities of fluids. He also urinates more than usual. In addition, his appetite may be markedly increased, despite the fact that he is losing weight.

These cardinal symptoms have a simple explanation. The diabetic person cannot use sugar and other foods properly. He wastes them. This explains his appetite and loss of weight. If the sugar content of the blood is too high, then sugar appears in the urine. The release of sugar by the kidneys is accompanied by a flow of excess water. This explains the increased thirst and excess urination.

This brings up a common misconception. People say, "I can't have diabetes because I don't have any sugar in my urine." There is normally a certain quantity of sugar in the bloodstream. This is used to supply energy to various parts of the body. The kidneys usually do not allow any of this sugar to filter out into the urine. This would be a waste of body foodstuffs. Only when the level of sugar in the blood reaches very high levels do the kidneys allow it to spill over into the urine. A person may have diabetes mellitus and an elevated blood sugar for some time before it thus appears in the urine.

The diagnosis of the disease rests primarily upon determining whether the level of sugar in the blood is higher than normal. Certainly, if sugar appears in the urine, this will prompt blood tests to confirm whether or not this represents diabetes mellitus. The presence of sugar in the urine does not necessarily indicate diabetes. In some persons, especially pregnant women, sugar may be spilled by the kidneys without a diabetic state being present. This is due to a temporary or permanent alteration in kidney function that may be unrelated to any type of diabetic process. The most exact way to determine the status of sugar management by the body is to check the level of sugar (glucose) in the blood before eating, and at various time intervals after eating ordinary foods or foods high in sugar content. If the pancreas is functioning properly and producing adequate amounts of insulin, then the sugar will rise to only certain levels, but if the insulin mechanism is defective, then the blood sugar level will become very high.

Medical science uses three main tools to treat diabetes mellitus—diet, insulin, and pills. The purpose of diet is twofold. First, we have seen that many people who develop diabetes are overweight. If they are in the group of individuals who develop maturity-onset diabetes, there is a good chance that their pancreas is still producing some insulin. The problem is just that their bodies are too big for the amount of insulin that the pancreas can produce. If a rigid diet reduces the weight of these persons to normal, then their own pancreas may be able to produce enough insulin to meet their individual requirements, and no further treatment will be necessary. Another way of stating this is that, in general, a large body requires more insulin each day than a small body. The person is capable of producing only so much insulin per day. If we shrink the body, his pancreas may still have enough action to take care of his needs. Furthermore, it is possible that the actual consumption of excess calories is putting a strain on the pancreas, and if this strain is removed, the pancreas will not be as likely to wear itself out prematurely.

The second reason for using a diet concerns juvenile diabetics and adults with more severe diabetes. These individuals are using insulin or pills to try to regulate their diabetic process. Medication is substituting for a natural body process. Let us stop here a moment and consider what the body normally does with insulin production. If a normal person eats a large meal, the pancreas is signaled to increase the amount of insulin put into the system. When the blood sugar returns to normal levels, the pancreas decreases the amount of insulin it is producing. If this same person then skips a meal, for example, lunch, the body recognizes that there is no elevation of blood sugar occurring at noontime. The pancreas does not release any additional insulin until the next food is consumed. The insulin normally produced does not stay in the body very long. In ten minutes about half of the insulin produced at any given moment disappears. The body can therefore constantly make adjustments throughout the day in response to eating. If a person eats ten times a day, then each of those times the pancreas can add insulin to the body. If the person eats only twice a day, then the body recognizes this and adds insulin only twice a day.

The case is entirely different for the diabetic who receives insulin injections. Most diabetics receive a single injection of insulin in the morning before breakfast. If his disease is difficult to regulate, he may also receive an injection of insulin before supper. The insulin will have an effect on his body for several hours. Several types of insulin are used, the chief difference between them being the duration of their action in the body after they have been administered.

There may be a period during the day when there is more injected insulin in the body than is required, and the blood sugar level may fall lower than normal. The body has several defensive measures that can be put into effect in this instance to correct the blood sugar temporarily. Primarily, the liver turns glycogen into glucose and amino acids, or proteins into glucose, to raise the blood sugar level to where it should be. If these measures are inadequate, the person will suffer what is termed an "insulin reaction." Initially the person feels weak and tremulous. He may feel hungry and start to perspire, as well as notice a rapid pulse. If nothing is done to counteract the reaction, he may lose consciousness. These symptoms are all usually reversed rapidly by eating sugar. Most diabetics who are taking insulin learn to carry some sugar cubes or candy in their pockets to have on hand at the first sign of any of these symptoms.

Insulin reactions usually occur if the diabetic skips a meal, or even if he eats a meal later than usual. We now can see why it is necessary for him to eat regularly spaced meals. Because of the possibility of excess insulin being present between meals, many physicians will prescribe midafternoon and bedtime snacks.

The amount of insulin a patient requires each day will depend upon how many calories he consumes and how active he is. If a person is very active, he will burn up more calories with his exercise. The amount of food he eats should be based on his activity, age (growing children require more calories), and weight. The doctor tries to match up the patient's calorie intake, insulin dose, and activity. The dosage of insulin is adjusted upward or downward in relation to the amount of glucose (sugar) that the doctor finds in the bloodstream at different times of the day. The diet can be increased if the person is losing too much weight or decreased if the weight is excessive. Once the formula has been determined for each patient, it is obvious that it must be adhered to; otherwise there will be periods of the day when his blood sugar is too high or too low for good health. It is easy to hold the insulin dosage constant, and if the person is conscientious, the daily calories can be held fairly constant too.

One problem that frequently arises is a variation in activity. During the week, a man may be relatively inactive on his job and then during the weekend he may expend much more energy doing work in his yard. If this man held his food intake and insulin dose constant, he would have a good chance of having an insulin reaction while working in his yard. In this situation, the patient would probably be instructed by his doctor either to take some extra food while working or to take a little less insulin that morning. Either of these measures would probably prevent an insulin reaction.

The diabetic diet will limit the amount of fat consumed daily. Since diabetics have a higher incidence of atherosclerosis than others, a dietary limitation of fat helps to control this factor.

A certain quantity of carbohydrates (sugars) will be included in the diet. Many persons erroneously believe that a diabetic cannot eat sugar. This would actually present an insurmountable problem, because many foods are converted to sugar by the body, and a diet completely lacking in carbohydrates would be unpalatable. In addition, the body requires a certain quantity of carbohydrates each day. If sugar is not available, body chemistry will rapidly become upset. On the other hand, the diet will certainly impose a limit. So much carbohydrate is beneficial; excess amounts will aggravate the diabetes.

We mentioned earlier that there were three main forms of treatment for diabetes mellitus—diet, insulin, and pills. Many persons with maturity-onset diabetes will require only a diet. Almost all persons with juvenile-onset diabetes require insulin. About one-third of patients with the maturity-onset category of diabetes will be able to use the pills. The balance that are not controlled with diet alone will have to use insulin.

The pills used are technically termed oral hypoglycemic agents. Hypoglycemic means acting to lower blood sugar. These agents are NOT insulin. No form of insulin can be taken orally. This point is emphasized because we have found patients who had so little knowledge of their diabetes and the oral drugs they were taking that they were doing dangerous things with the medicine. They thought the pills were a direct substitute for insulin, and instead of taking the prescribed number of tablets a day, they were taking extra pills whenever they cheated on their diet. They thought that the extra pill would take care of the dessert or other sweet that they ate. This is not the case, and they were risking developing a low blood sugar hours after they took the pills.

There are two categories of oral hypoglycemic drugs. The first category is comprised of tolbutamide (Orinase®), chlorpropamide (Diabinese®), acetohexamide (Dymelor®), and tolazamide (Tolinase®). This group of drugs apparently acts primarily by stimulating the pancreas to produce more insulin. The reason that these drugs usually are not effective in the juvenile-onset type of diabetic is that shortly after this type of diabetes develops, the pancreas is completely emptied of insulin and stops producing it. The dosage used varies between patients, and some individuals may take one tablet a day, while others may take the medicine several times a day. It is important to emphasize that these drugs stimulate the pancreas during many hours of the day, and low blood sugar reactions can occur just as they do in persons who are taking insulin injections. It is therefore important not to skip meals when these drugs are used. The temptation to skip meals occurs more often when persons go on sporadic diets to lose weight.

The diet is just as important here as it is for the diabetic using insulin. Obesity must be controlled. The penalty for cheating on the diet when oral hypoglycemic drugs are used is the possibility of eventually requiring a shift over to insulin injections. Between 20 and 30 percent of patients whose diabetes is initially controlled with the oral drugs will gradually fail to respond to the drugs over a period of months to years. The failure rate is probably higher among those persons who continue to overtax their pancreas by excess ingestion of carbohydrates (sugars).

The second group of oral hypoglycemic drugs contains only one agent. This drug is phenformin (DBI®). This drug has a different mechanism of action, one that is not well understood. It does not stimulate the pancreas to produce more insulin, a fact we know because this drug will work in some diabetics who have had their pancreas removed surgically. The drug probably has some direct action on the body cells to assist them in utilizing glucose (sugar). The drug is somewhat limited in its usefulness because of its side effects. Phenformin is frequently used in conjunction with one of the other oral hypoglycemic drugs or injected insulin to help achieve smoother control of the diabetes.

A ten-year clinical study comparing the use of diet, oral hypoglycemic drugs, and insulin in the treatment of mild diabetics prompted comment from the U.S. Food and Drug Administration in 1970. The FDA recommended that diabetic patients who could not control their disease by diet alone should be treated with insulin in preference to the oral drugs. The recommendation was made because this study had revealed that the patients taking one of the oral drugs had a higher number of deaths due to diseases of the heart and blood vessels than those diabetics in the study who were treated with diet alone or diet and insulin.

A great deal of controversy arose over both the study and the FDA stands, with medical experts taking both sides of the argument. With the discovery of the oral drugs to treat diabetes, many diabetics and their physicians were lulled into a false sense of security, but it has become apparent that many diabetic patients were using the pills as a substitute for weight loss and a diabetic diet. Many persons with mild diabetes would not require any form of treatment if they were able to reduce their body weight to normal. One result of the oral drug controversy is a reaffirmation that the ideal manner to treat maturity-onset diabetes mellitus is to reduce the body weight to normal. If this measure fails to control the diabetic process, then the physician and his patient decide upon what form of additional treatment is indicated—insulin or oral drugs. The decision should be based on a consideration of all the factors, including the potential risk of each form of treatment.

One of the more alarming acute complications of diabetes mellitus is the development of diabetic acidosis, or diabetic coma. This occurs usually in persons who have severe, undiagnosed diabetes, or in known diabetics who skip their insulin or develop an infection or other serious illness. The term diabetic acidosis refers to the situation in which there is inadequate insulin in the body, and as a result the blood sugar becomes very elevated and body fats and proteins are broken down and circulate in abnormal amounts. These fat and protein substances interfere with normal body function and actually poison the body. The person so affected usually is nauseated, vomits, may have abdominal pain, feels weak and dried out, and eventually may lapse into a coma.

A confusing point occurs soon after the development of diabetic acidosis with the person who is taking insulin. He feels nauseated or may vomit, and he realizes that he will not be able to eat as usual that day. Reasoning that if he is not able to eat, and if he takes his usual amount of insulin he will have an insulin reaction, the person usually skips his insulin or takes a smaller amount than usual. At this particular time, the person actually requires more insulin than usual.

Diabetic acidosis can also occur in a person who is taking oral hypoglycemic agents. He, too, may be confronted with the problem of what to do about his pills when he knows he will be unable to eat. The oral hypoglycemic agents are of no value in diabetic acidosis, and this person requires insulin at this time. The key to the solution of the problem lies in contacting the doctor. If the case is severe enough, the patient will have to be hospitalized, administered large amounts of insulin, and given intravenous feedings of water and salts.

An infection in some part of the body may be the trigger that initiates the process of diabetic acidosis. For this reason, diabetics with serious infections are frequently hospitalized so that their insulin can be adjusted as necessary to try to prevent acidosis from developing.

The diabetic process has another serious complication. Over a number of years, diabetics develop a deterioration of very small blood vessels. This small blood vessel disease eventually results in changes in the eyes and the kidneys. In the eye, small blood vessels leak blood cells into the tissues of the eye. Over a time this can cause a gradual loss of vision. Cataracts occur more often than usual in diabetics, and glaucoma can suddenly develop and mar vision.

In the kidneys, the process is less evident. The formation of urine is dependent upon water and wastes filtering through small blood vessels. Some of these tiny vessels in the kidneys of a diabetic may become blocked or distorted so that the filtering function is at the same time decreased and less selective. One of the early signs is a leakage of albumin or protein into the urine in abnormal amounts. The result is frequently hypertension (high blood pressure) and uremia. Uremia is chronic poisoning from waste products that are usually eliminated by the kidneys.

It is felt that all of these complications of diabetes can be slowed or prevented by control of the disease state through proper diet and medication.

16
Hypertension—
High Blood Pressure

Hypertension—high blood pressure—is a serious health problem in the United States. It is estimated that 20,000,000 Americans have this disease. Regrettable as the facts may be, at least half of this number are not aware that they have high blood pressure.

Fortunately for all of us today, high blood pressure can be controlled in the majority of instances with drugs and surgical procedures. A person who develops hypertension can look forward to a near normal life expectancy if he follows instructions and takes care of himself. One of the biggest problems in regard to hypertension is identifying the individuals who have the disease. Since high blood pressure usually does not produce any symptoms unless a complication of the disease occurs, the average hypertensive person may be free of symptoms for years, even if he is not receiving treatment. The solution to the detection problem is simple: everyone should have a blood pressure checkup once a year. This is one of the many reasons for periodic health examinations.

The undetected hypertensive person faces the same risks that all hypertensive patients faced before the new anti-hypertensive drugs were introduced during the early 1950s. Previously, about 45 percent of all the deaths caused by diseases of the heart and blood vessels could be traced to hypertension. Furthermore, a person with hypertension had about a 60 percent chance that he would die of some heart complication, especially heart failure.

High blood pressure has several effects on the heart. It makes the heart work harder to circulate the blood throughout the body. As a result, the heart enlarges and may wear out prematurely. Frequently it leads to heart failure, with the heart being unable to pump an adequate amount of blood. A second important effect of hypertension is to accelerate and aggravate the development of atherosclerosis in the coronary arteries. This is the process that eventually leads to heart attacks or myocardial infarctions and most strokes.

Before we describe high blood pressure, let us examine what normal blood pressure is and what it means. When we use the term "blood pressure," we are referring to the pressure of the blood inside the arteries of the body. It is measured with a blood pressure cuff and a stethoscope. The blood pressure cuff is constructed of cloth, inside of which is an inflatable rubber bladder. The cuff is wrapped securely around either upper arm. Then, with a rubber bulb, air is pumped into the bladder. The patient feels the cuff tighten around the arm. During the measurement the operator observes a gauge attached to the cuff and calibrated in millimeters of mercury. The stethoscope (a listening and amplifying device) is placed over the brachial artery at the crease in the arm.

The cuff is inflated until the pressure registered on the gauge exceeds the blood pressure, indicated by cessation of the pulse sound in the stethoscope. The pressure in the cuff is then slowly released and the needle on the gauge starts to drop. The operator then listens closely. At some point he begins to hear a "thump, thump, thump." The point on the gauge where a sound is first heard is the systolic blood pressure, the pressure when the heart contracts. The sounds continue, as the cuff air pressure is released, and finally cease. The lower point on the gauge where sounds finally stop is called the diastolic blood pressure, the pressure when the heart dilates. Thus, if a person has a blood pressure of 130/70, the number 130 is the systolic pressure, and 70 represents the diastolic blood pressure.

Five principal factors determine the blood pressure. An alteration in any one of these may produce a change in the blood pressure if some countermeasure is not taken by the body to maintain a normal pressure. An elaborate system of regulatory mechanisms exists in the body that is capable of making various adjustments. The five primary factors are as follows.

1. First is the pumping action of the heart. With each heartbeat, a certain amount of blood is sent out into the arteries of the body. If the heart is weakened, as by a heart attack, the amount of blood pumped may decrease below normal, and as a result, the blood pressure may fall below normal.

2. The second factor is the volume of blood in the arteries. If a person has a hemorrhage and loses blood, his blood pressure may fall. If this same person inadvertently receives too much blood by transfusion, his blood pressure may rise higher than normal.

3. An increase in blood viscosity (thickness) can elevate the blood pressure. This situation occurs in persons who have excessive red blood cells (polycythemia). The blood does not flow as easily as it should, and this produces an increased resistance to flow that is transmitted as an elevation of pressure.

4. An easier factor to understand is the elasticity of the arteries. These blood vessels have large amounts of elastic tissue in their walls, and when the heart pumps out a charge of blood, the blood vessels tend to expand to absorb some of the thrust. Between heartbeats, the blood vessels contract to their normal size. This contraction of the arteries between heartbeats is a factor that tends to smooth out the blood flow, and is also a reason that the diastolic blood pressure does not fall to zero. The elastic tissue in the walls of the larger arteries may wear out prematurely or be destroyed by deposits of atherosclerosis. As a result, in some people, especially in the older age groups, this rebound action of the arteries is lost, most often resulting in an elevation of the systolic blood pressure and possibly in a reduction of the diastolic pressure. Thus a man of 40 may have a blood pressure of 140/80, and when he becomes 60 his blood pressure could be 160/65. This pressure, 160/65, is normal for a person at that age. If any measures are taken to reduce the systolic pressure, certain parts of his body may not get adequate blood flow.

5. The last important factor governing blood pressure is the resistance encountered by the blood as it flows into the smaller arteries. The small arteries in all parts of the body have the capacity to change their diameter, or caliber. This change is under the influence of a particular part of the nervous system (sympathetic nervous system) and certain hormones (primarily adrenaline). If the small arteries nar-

row themselves, the blood pressure is elevated. If the diameter of these vessels is increased, the blood pressure will tend to fall. This may be better appreciated if we visualize a tube of tooth paste or airplane glue. If we put a pinpoint hole in the end of the tube and then try to squeeze out the contents of the tube, we have to squeeze hard to get any results. If, on the other hand, we put a much larger hole in the end of the tube and squeeze, the contents pour out. This is the factor of resistance.

The next important question is, what is normal blood pressure? Blood pressure varies with the age of the person in question. Infants and children have a lower blood pressure than adolescents or adults. We have just seen how a loss of elasticity in blood vessels can produce a relatively high pressure in older persons. Opinion varies greatly among experts in the field as to the point at which high blood pressure is considered to be present in a person in the 20- to 60-year age group. Many doctors would consider a blood pressure above 150/90 in this age group to be abnormal, while some doctors would accept up to 160/95 as within normal limits. Certainly when the diastolic pressure is over 100, few would dispute the presence of hypertension. In general, the most important component of the blood pressure is the diastolic pressure, the bottom number. If peripheral resistance (small artery narrowing) is greater than normal, it elevates primarily the diastolic pressure, and most cases of significant hypertension are due to an elevated peripheral resistance.

A recent study has shown that in older persons, an elevated systolic pressure is of definite concern. The study covered 5,192 men and women in Framingham, Massachusetts over a period of sixteen years. During this period of time, 142 persons developed heart failure. In 75 percent of the cases of heart failure which occurred in the age range of from 30 to 62 years, hypertension was the underlying cause. There was no difference between diastolic hypertension and systolic hypertension as a causative force. In other words, although the systolic pressure rises with age, an unusual elevation should be treated to prevent the occurrence of heart failure.

An interesting point about blood pressure is that each individual's blood pressure varies from moment to moment. While recording the pressure in the arm of a normal person, the readings may vary from 120/70 to 140/80 as the readings are repeated over and over again. A person's blood pressure will tend to be lower in the morning when he awakens, and it will rise as he becomes active during the day. Exercise and emotional excitement will both invariably elevate it. As a result of these facts, each person will have a range of pressures during the day, and if most of them are within normal limits, there is no problem. If, on the other hand, several readings are found to be above normal, then the person may be in the early stages of hypertension. This is often a difficult point to determine. Is the patient just excited by the blood pressure examination or does he persistently have an elevated pressure? For this reason, doctors will frequently request that a number of determinations be made of a person's pressure if there is any question about one or two individual readings.

When a person develops hypertension, it is usually a gradual process. He does not awaken one morning with hypertension. The pressures gradually increase over a period of time, leading to a constantly elevated pressure. There is no difficulty in making the diagnosis at this point. The doubtful cases are those that may be temporarily elevated due to stress or those which represent the early stages of hypertension.

In some ways the hypertensive process represents an accentuation of normal processes. For example, a person may have a pressure of 120/72 when he is resting, and then have an elevation of 150/85 when he is exercising. This is a response within the range of normal. A certain hypertensive patient had a blood pressure before treatment that ranged from 180/100 to 200/110. With medication over a period of time, his blood pressure had been reduced to 160/90. As I was checking his blood pressure, he began to tell me about an automobile accident that he had been involved in the previous week. As he talked, his pressure rose from 170/100 to 230/120! I asked him to think about something else and continued to observe his blood pressure. Within a minute it fell to 160/90.

Such sudden fluctuations in blood pressure are probably due mainly to the activity of the sympathetic nervous system, an automatic regulatory system with its origins in the brain. Under normal conditions it serves a very useful purpose. For example, when a person suddenly stands up after lying in bed for some time, he ordinarily does not feel much different. In making that change in his body position though, if something had not happened to increase the blood flow to his brain, his brain might have been momentarily robbed of blood by the effect of gravity. In the normal person, a part of the brain that keeps track of the body's position signaled another part of the brain that the person was going to stand up. This second portion of the brain then sent a message through the sympathetic nervous system to his small blood vessels. These blood vessels, in turn, narrowed themselves to temporarily raise the blood pressure to ensure that the brain received a constant supply of blood.

When the sympathetic nervous system is slow or sluggish,

suddenly standing up from a lying or seated position produces a sensation of dizziness or giddiness for a few seconds. This is called postural vertigo. It is due to a momentary lack of blood flow to the brain. Similarly, the brain signals the blood pressure through this system when the person is exercising or is excited. The effect is to raise the blood pressure. In a way, this system resembles the thermostat in a house that regulates the temperature inside the house. Some authorities believe that certain types of hypertension are due to a fault in this "thermostat" that regulates the blood pressure.

It is interesting that some persons who have had hypertension for several years, and in whom the blood pressure has been adequately controlled with drugs, eventually develop normal blood pressures again and can stop using any medication. It is felt that in these fortunate persons the thermostat or barostat in the brain that regulates the blood pressure has been reset at a lower reading due to the influence of the drugs over a sufficient time.

When a physician is confronted with a patient with hypertension, his first reaction is not to reach for the prescription pad and begin to write, but to ask himself, "Why does this person have an elevated blood pressure, and can the cause of this problem be eliminated?" In about ten percent of persons with high blood pressure, there is a specific reason for their hypertension. In the remaining 90 percent of hypertensives the cause is not known, and this group is labeled with the diagnostic term "essential hypertension." This term defines by not defining. It simply means that not enough is known about the blood pressure mechanism to understand why this group of people has a persistent elevation of pressure.

The best mechanism available to help decide which type

of hypertension a patient has is the physical examination, during which the doctor looks for clues that might indicate that a curable type of hypertension is present. The curable forms of hypertension that the physician will be looking for are anemia (inadequate quantity or quality of red blood cells) and hyperthyroidism (over-active thyroid gland), both of which produce an elevation of the systolic pressure that is corrected when the basic disease is adequately treated. Combined systolic and diastolic hypertension is found in persons with polycythemia (excess numbers of red blood cells). It is also found in people with certain types of brain tumors. Brain tumors can usually be suspected by abnormal findings that are encountered in a routine physical examination.

A form of hypertension often found in younger persons is due to a coarctation of the aorta, the large blood vessel that leaves the heart to carry blood to the body. In the condition of coarctation, there is an abnormally narrowed segment of the aorta shortly after its origin. This constriction produces hypertension in the aorta and its branches that arise before the constriction is encountered. Beyond the area of constriction the blood pressure is normal, or even lower than usual. The branches that supply blood to the arms are usually under high pressure, while the legs will have a normal or low pressure. This fact facilitates making the diagnosis. The blood pressure is recorded first in the arms and then in the legs. If there is a difference, a coarctation is suggested. A murmur (abnormal sound) is frequently heard over the chest near the area of constriction. This form of hypertension can be corrected by surgery. The narrowed segment of aorta is removed and the normal size ends of the vessel are sewn together again.

Certain tumors of the adrenal glands can produce hypertension that is surgically curable. Either the tumors or the entire gland can be removed and the hypertension will disappear. The trick here is to diagnose the presence of the tumor. One type of tumor is called a pheochromocytoma. This tumor arises in the center of the adrenal gland and produces abnormally large amounts of epinephrine and norepinephrine. These substances are similar to Adrenalin®. Adrenalin, incidentally, is the trademark name of commercially produced epinephrine. This type of tumor can produce either a sustained hypertension or recurrent episodes of hypertension with periods of normal blood pressure in between. The episodic form is usually associated with recurrent headaches. an awareness of the heart beating abnormally fast, and marked perspiration. The excess epinephrine is passed out in the urine, and the disease can therefore be detected by collecting a large sample of urine (usually over a 24-hour period) and examining the urine for abnormal amounts of epinephrine.

A second type of adrenal tumor produces a disease called Cushing's syndrome, which has associated hypertension. This tumor produces abnormal amounts of cortisone. The person with this problem usually has a round face and a hump of fat under the skin of the back near the neck, which has been given the descriptive term "buffalo hump." These tumors can also be detected by measuring a 24-hour sample of urine for the presence of cortisone.

A final type of adrenal tumor produces excess amounts of a hormone named aldosterone. This hormone normally controls the body's sodium (salt) balance, but when it is produced excessively, salt is retained and the blood pressure becomes secondarily elevated. Diagnosis is more difficult with this type of tumor, but the physician can suspect its presence by measuring the amount of sodium bicarbonate and potassium in the bloodstream.

The kidneys are known to play a role in the development of hypertension in certain individuals. Persons who have chronic infection in one or both kidneys (pyelonephritis) will frequently eventually develop high blood pressure. There is also a condition known as glomerulonephritis that may result in hypertension. This disease is a chronic inflammation of the kidney tissue. It may be initiated by a streptococcal infection in some other part of the body, which is followed by kidney inflamation due to an allergic reaction on the part of the kidney to a poison elaborated by the streptococcus. These two diseases are very common, and they are not among the types of hypertension that are curable unless the situation is so extreme that a kidney transplant is warranted. In such a case the accompanying hypertension may disappear following transplant.

The exact mechanism by which the kidney contributes to or causes the development of hypertension in these diseases is unknown. But an interesting mechanism has been uncovered in the case of a single kidney that has a deficient blood supply. The deficient supply is usually due to a narrowing of the renal artery (the blood vessel that supplies the kidney) as a result of atherosclerosis or from a band of scar tissue that narrows one segment of the artery. In response to less than normal blood flow, the affected kidney produces a substance called renin. This acts upon another substance that circulates in the bloodstream to form a chemical called angiotensin. This material stimulates the adrenal glands to produce excess amounts of aldosterone, which, as we have seen, can cause salt retention and hypertension. This type of problem (a single kidney with inadequate blood supply) is frequently curable by surgery. The affected artery is either replaced by a graft (artificial blood vessel) or the kidney is removed. Abnormalities that appear in special x-rays of the kidneys (intravenous pyelogram) indicate the diagnosis.

If the physical examination and laboratory tests that are performed on a person with recently recognized hypertension do not establish the presence of any of the problems described above, he is considered to be in the 90 percent group with essential hypertension. The primary goal in the management of these persons is to control the blood pressure with various drugs to prevent the high blood pressure from eventually damaging the body.

The untreated person with persistent hypertension faces complications involving his heart, brain, and kidneys. The time necessary for hypertension to produce these complications is variable. Some may have hypertension for years without any serious complications, while others may develop an accelerated phase of the hypertension and have serious problems within a matter of months. Actually, any untreated hypertensive is susceptible to a sudden acceleration in the severity of his disease. This accelerated phase is called malignant hypertension. There is no relationship to cancer; the term malignant merely signifies that the process is virulent and getting worse.

The cardiac response to hypertension is usually an enlargement of the heart, especially the left ventricle, the main pumping chamber. There is usually an accelerated development of atherosclerosis of the coronary arteries, and a heart attack or angina pectoris may occur. Eventually the heart may weaken, and the person will then develop heart failure, with shortness of breath and swelling of the body.

In a person with hypertension, the blood vessels that supply the brain may intermittently narrow (vasospasm) with the resultant lack of adequate blood flow to parts of the brain. This may produce periods of confusion, actual unconsciousness, or intermittent periods of paralysis of one side of the body. The arteries usually also develop increased degrees of atherosclerosis, and this process may lead to the permanent occlusion of one of the vessels or to its rupture with bleeding into the brain. These events produce strokes, with paralysis or death.

The small blood vessels that lie inside the kidneys can be affected by prolonged or severe hypertension. The response in these blood vessels is to deposit a coating on the inside of the vessel, which results in the vessels becoming narrower than normal. The kidneys then suffer from a lack of blood flow. This eventually produces gradual death of parts of the kidney, with ensuing kidney failure or uremia. As uremia develops in the hypertensive person, we frequently see that they lose weight and their appetite. They often become anemic, and edema or swelling of the lower parts of the body develops.

We mentioned earlier that with proper treatment, a hypertensive patient may have a near normal life span. This is particularly true if his problem is detected before any complications occur.

Prior to 1950 there were very few effective techniques for treating hypertension. Sedatives were used to help lower the pressure in mild cases, but those people with malignant hypertension had an inauspicious future. The death rate in malignant hypertension took 80 percent of those so affected in the first year. Severe salt restriction helped some people. This was the era of the rice diet, or low salt diet.

Then the *Rauwolfia serpentina,* or Indian snake root, entered the scene. Derivatives of this plant are still some of the principal agents used today to control blood pressure. A short time later the first of the modern diuretic drugs appeared. A variety of different diuretic drugs is now available. They act primarily by removing excess salt from the body. As a result, salt restriction is usually not necessary in the hypertensive patient. Additional drugs have been developed that block the blood pressure mechanism at different levels in the body. Agents may work primarily on the brain, the sympathetic nervous system, the small arteries of the body, or the kidneys. The stronger agents have side effects that may hinder their use in certain persons, but such a wide range of effective drugs are in existence today that the vast majority of hypertensive patients can now be adequately managed by one or more drugs.

17

Strokes

Many people confuse heart attacks and strokes. A heart attack or myocardial infarct is actually the death of a piece of the heart due to an interruption in the blood supply to that particular part of the heart. A stroke is produced by an interruption in the blood supply to a portion of the brain. The result is brain damage and abnormal function of some part of the body, such as paralysis of an arm or leg, loss of vision, or the inability to concentrate or speak.

The brain ordinarily receives 20 percent of the total blood supply pumped by the heart. It is dependent upon an adequate blood supply to function and to stay alive. If a person's heart stops beating temporarily, he may lose consciousness in 10 to 20 seconds, because certain parts of the brain do not function normally without fresh blood and oxygen. The brain of animals has been found to die within three minutes after the brain blood supply was interrupted. These examples concern the brain as a whole. If the blood supply to one part of the brain is interrupted for only a few seconds, that part will temporarily cease to function. If there is a permanent blockage of the same vessel, that particular part of the brain will die.

Before we proceed with a discussion of strokes it may be well to consider a little bit of the anatomy of the brain and nervous system. The appearance of the brain in some ways resembles a mushroom. The cap of the mushroom represents the cortex or gray matter of the brain. In this area are located the brain cells that are responsible for our thought processes, smell, speech, sight, and muscular movements. The wire-like connections between the different functioning parts of the brain and between the brain and different parts of the body are called nerves. The stem of the mushroom corresponds to the nerves. The main "trunk line" of wires that connects the brain to the body is the spinal cord. This is connected to the base of the brain, runs down through the backbone (vertebral column), and sends off branch nerves to various parts of the body.

Different systems throughout the body pick up pieces of information and relay them to the brain for handling. The eyes and ears and the senses of taste and smell are examples of these sensing devices. We also have special sensing organs in our skin to detect temperature and pain.

Here is an example of the function of the different components of this system. When we burn a finger with a match, the sensation of heat and pain is detected by nerve endings in the finger. A message is sent via a nerve through the spinal cord to our brain. The sensation is interpreted by a portion of the brain, which flashes a signal to that portion of the cortex that controls the muscles of the arm. This segment of the cortex then relays a message back through the spinal cord to the nerves in the arm. The result is a motion to jerk our arm away from the painful flame.

The blood supply of the brain is such that alternate paths of blood flow are provided in case a major artery is obstructed. Four main arteries supply blood to the brain. They originate from the aorta very close to the heart. Two large carotid arteries course up from the aorta through the front of the neck toward the brain, and two smaller vertebral arteries pass up the vertebral bones in the neck. All four arteries enter the bottom of the skull near the base of the brain. Here the arteries have a common communication with each other, much like a traffic circle, before they go to different portions of the brain. This circle, called the circle of Willis, is a very important communication. If blood in one of the arteries is blocked in the neck before it reaches the circle of Willis, it will still flow into the brain as originally intended. The other three arteries pick up the deficit at the circle of Willis and shunt blood to all portions of the brain.

A second area of intercommunication among the different arteries is created by the small end branches that run over the surface of the brain. The end branches from one major artery communicate with the end branches of another major artery. Therefore, if a major vessel is blocked beyond the communication point at the circle of Willis, there is still a chance that the brain will be able to get adequate nourishment via a shunt of blood through the small arteries on the brain's surface.

We mentioned previously that a stroke was due to some portion of the brain tissue losing its ability to function. This is typically caused by the death of part of the brain tissue, caused, in turn, by interruption of the normal blood flow to that part. In the majority of patients who have had a stroke, the basic problem with the involved artery is atherosclerosis. This is the same atherosclerosis that we discussed previously in relation to heart attacks. The details that were discussed relative to the changes that occur in the arteries and the factors that predispose a person to the development of atherosclerosis are the same whether the disease affects arteries in the heart or in the brain.

An artery supplying blood to the brain can be involved with any one of three different processes that will result in its blood flow being interrupted: the artery can be blocked by a thrombus, blocked by an embolus, or the artery can rupture.

A thrombus is a blood clot that forms inside a portion of the artery. The blood clot usually forms on a patch of atherosclerosis. The exact reason for the clot forming at any particular moment is unknown, but it could occur as a result of decreased blood flow passing by a narrowed segment of artery. The decreased flow could be caused by a temporary fall in blood pressure (such as might occur in association with a heart attack), or by a further narrowing of the artery in response to elevated blood pressure to protect tissues further down the line from the stress induced by the higher pressure.

An embolus is a piece of free floating material inside an artery that eventually flows into a small enough vessel to get stuck in it. The embolus may be a piece of atherosclerotic patch that has become detached. It is most often a piece of a blood clot. The inside of the heart is the most common site of the original clot that embolizes to the brain. The commonest reason for blood clots forming inside the heart is atrial fibrillation, the condition wherein the atria are quivering instead of regularly beating. A small side pocket of the atria, called the auricle, can trap blood and form blood clots under this condition. Blood clots may also form on the inside of the ventricles of the heart as a consequence of myocardial infarctions.

Finally, an artery may rupture. The blood that leaks outside the torn artery presses on normal brain tissue and destroys it. If the hemorrhage is massive, it may destroy so much brain tissue that the person cannot survive. If the torn vessel clots and seals itself off, the damage may be small enough for the person to survive. Rupture of a small artery in the brain and brain hemorrhages are more prone to occur in persons with hypertension. The high blood pressure puts a strain on the blood vessels, and eventually one of them may break.

In a study made in Framingham, Massachusetts, over a period of 14 years, over 5,000 persons in good health between the ages of 30 and 62 years of age were observed in order to determine the natural occurrence of various types of heart and blood vessel diseases. One of the results of this study was the determination that 85 percent of all persons who developed strokes had hypertension. Of interest is the fact that the elevated blood pressure was usually present for many years before the strokes occurred and usually caused cardiac damage. The damage manifested itself in the form of heart failure or myocardial infarctions. We just discussed the manner in which a heart attack could induce the development of a stroke, either through a lowered blood pressure or by an embolization of a blood clot that formed inside the heart. Heart failure would predispose a person to developing a stroke by the mechanism of decreased blood flow and a lowered blood pressure. Arteries narrowed by atherosclerosis would tend to develop clots in the presence of a sluggish blood flow.

The obvious conclusion that can be drawn from this study is that the detection and control of hypertension in its early stages will decrease death and disability from diseases of the heart and blood vessels.

A stroke can occur without complete occlusion of one of the main arteries that supplies the brain during an episode of *hypo*tension, or low blood pressure. The mechanism is as follows: if the pressure in the entire blood vessel system falls below a certain critical point, body organs will not receive adequate oxygen and food. The brain is the organ of the body that is most sensitive to inadequate blood flow, so it is usually the organ that is damaged first during an episode of hypotension. If blood flow is very low or absent, and if the condition persists for more than a few minutes, the entire brain will die. A stroke could occur, however, if the blood flow were below normal but sufficient to prevent death of the entire brain. In this case, if the person had an area of narrowing in one of the main arteries in his brain, the brain tissue beyond the point of narrowing might not receive enough oxygen to stay alive, but the brain as a whole would be able to survive.

Low blood pressure can occur in a variety of situations. The association of a stroke following hypotension is most often seen in myocardial infarctions. In some persons who have a heart attack, the heart is not able to pump as much blood as it should for a period of time. This causes a lowering of the blood pressure that could result in a stroke by the mechanism described above. Approximately 20 percent of persons who suffer a stroke have had a recent heart attack. If the stroke alters the patient's ability to speak or to remember, the physician caring for him may not know that the patient had been suffering from a chest pain. For this reason, all persons who have had a stroke are also examined with an electrocardiogram and blood tests to determine whether or not heart damage is also present.

When they operate on elderly persons, surgeons and anesthetists are particularly careful to avoid a complicating stroke through a drop in blood pressure. A final common cause of low blood pressure and strokes in the elderly is massive bleeding, anywhere within or from the body. Bleeding ulcers or accidents with severe hemorrhage could thus precipitate strokes.

Any of the major arteries of the brain or one of their branches can be obstructed by a stroke process. The variety of consequences is almost infinite. A very tiny branch that supplies a less important part of the brain could be occluded with no resultant symptoms. If the area of the brain that controls speech or the use of the left arm is involved, then the patient will have difficulty speaking or using that arm.

Physicians are usually able to determine the area of the brain and the blood vessel involved in a stroke by the symptoms that develop. Furthermore, it is frequently possible to differentiate between a stroke due to a brain hemorrhage, an embolism, and a thrombosis. A patient with an embolism has a sudden occlusion of a blood vessel and develops stroke symptoms as quickly as if he had been shot. One moment he is active and about his daily affairs, and the next moment he is unable to walk or speak. In some fortunate people, the embolus may fragment and the smaller pieces then float downstream. If the particles block unimportant vessels, the stroke may rapidly clear up. The person with a cerebral hemorrhage will usually develop his symptoms progressively over a period of a few hours as the blood continues to escape from the ruptured vessel. Strokes due to a thrombosis typically develop in a "stuttering" manner. The person usually experiences weakness of an arm or leg for a few minutes repeatedly over a period of hours, days, or weeks before the paralysis becomes complete.

Examination of the cerebrospinal fluid is a further help in

differentiating the various causes of strokes. The brain and the spinal cord are bathed by a clear liquid that freely circulates through and around them. If a patient has a brain hemorrhage, blood usually leaks into this spinal fluid and its presence can be detected. Persons who have sustained a stroke due to a thrombosis or an embolism seldom have associated bleeding into the brain or cerebrospinal fluid. A sample of this fluid is easily obtained by a needle puncture low in the back.

The primary concern in regard to strokes is in attempting to prevent them. Once a portion of the brain has died, nothing can be done to restore function in that area. Other parts of the brain may be trained to take over some of the functions that had been served by the damaged area, but the results are less than perfect. In rehabilitation, the patient's disabilities are evaluated, and an attempt is made to retrain other parts of the body to compensate for the losses. Several months may be required to achieve maximum results in speech therapy, walking, and self care.

Hypertension is controlled to prevent further strokes. In the case of the person with the "stuttering" thrombosis, the control of high blood pressure may prevent the final stroke if the patient seeks help early enough. Persons who have suffered a stroke due to an embolism are usually given anticoagulants to attempt to prevent a subsequent embolism. These drugs are also frequently prescribed for persons who are identified as being in the early stages of a thrombotic stroke. They are not used, of course, in persons who have a cerebral hemorrhage. They would only aggravate the problem.

Surgery can sometimes be very helpful in reducing the likelihood of a stroke. Patches of atherosclerosis and blood clots can be removed in the arteries that pass through the neck en route to the brain, but surgery is difficult and seldom attempted on arteries in the skull. Surgery is not attempted if the patient has already had a stroke. In this circumstance, the brain tissue has already died, and correction of the blood supply will not reverse the brain damage. Surgery may be helpful, however, for the person with the stuttering thrombotic stroke who is having warning periods of temporary paralysis if it is performed before the final complete stroke occurs.

The following case demonstrates some features of the thrombotic stroke. Harold awoke one morning and noted that his right arm felt numb. As he got out of bed, he shook the arm and rubbed it with his left hand and shortly afterward the arm felt normal again. He quickly forgot the matter. The following morning while he was eating breakfast he spilled coffee on himself as he was raising the cup to his lips with his right hand. He was able to put the cup back in the saucer, but he found it difficult to move the fingers of his right hand. A couple of minutes later these strange happenings ended, and he was able to use his hand properly. Over the following days he noted that intermittently his right hand and arm felt numb. The following week he noticed that something was wrong with his vision. He closed one eye and then the other, and much to his dismay, he found that he could not see out of his left eye. He called his family doctor and arranged to see him that afternoon. The vision returned in his left eye before he was due to see the doctor, and Harold felt a bit sheepish as he described these strange events to his physician. His doctor reassured him that he was wise in reporting the symptoms. He told Harold further that he suspected that he might have trouble with his left carotid artery. He explained that this artery supplied the major blood vessel to his left eye. The carotid artery then went up to the brain and supplied an area of his brain that controlled his right arm and leg. The symptoms that Harold had experienced were frequently warning signs that a thrombosis was occurring in this artery.

Harold was referred that afternoon to an ophthalmologist (eye doctor) who performed various tests. The most important test was ophthalmodynamometry, the measurement of the artery blood pressure in each eye. This test showed that the pressure in the left eye was lower than that in the right eye. The doctor felt for pulsations in Harold's neck and was able to detect the pulsations of the carotid arteries. He told Harold that the pulsation in the left artery was weaker than that in the right. These findings were interpreted for Harold by the doctor to indicate that there probably was a narrowing in his left carotid artery that was responsible for his recent symptoms.

Harold was immediately admitted to the hospital. The next morning he was taken to the x-ray department, where carotid arteriograms were performed. These are special x-rays of the blood vessels in the neck. They definitely established a narrowing of the left carotid artery in an area of his neck that could be reached by surgery. In an operation later that afternoon, the surgeon was not able to remove the material that partially blocked the artery, but he did assure an adequate blood flow to the brain by putting in a segment of artificial blood vessel that bypassed the obstruction.

Harold had an uneventful recovery and was saved the ordeal of awakening one morning with a paralyzed right arm and leg.

18

Can I Prevent A Heart Attack?

There is every reason to believe that you can avoid having a heart attack, just as you can avoid contracting cholera in India or tuberculosis in Peru.

Avoiding cholera is easier, so we'll start there. Before traveling to India, you would be immunized against the disease. Since cholera is mainly spread through food contaminated by the feces of infected persons, during your travels through the continent you would avoid drinking water from any questionable source. You would also eat meals only at those establishments catering to travelers, and thus you would have some assurance that the foods served to you have been prepared with more than the customary, local care.

There is no definite immunization against tuberculosis, but it is now well known that the disease is most often contracted in those areas where people live and work in very close contact with each other. If you avoid visiting slums and stay away from crowds of local people, you will greatly diminish your chances of coming in contact with the infection. Furthermore, your general state of health is usually somewhat of a safeguard as the disease is much more likely to affect persons chronically ill or malnourished. Tuberculosis exists today only in those areas of the world where people still live in crowded, primitive conditions and where other forms of disease and malnutrition exist.

Coronary heart disease, the disease that causes heart attacks, exists in the United States today in epidemic proportions. The problem has been likened to an epidemic because every American male has one chance in five that he will have a heart attack before he reaches the age of sixty. Women's chances are two to three times better, but they are still at high risk.

Just as tuberculosis was controlled in the United States during the early part of this century by an improvement in living and working conditions, sanitation, and appropriate medical care, coronary heart disease can be controlled. This can be done on an individual as well as a community basis once the factors that are responsible for the epidemic are generally recognized and dealt with.

The single most important factor that is responsible for our developing premature hardening of the arteries and heart attacks is diet. In the past twenty years, evidence has accumulated from many sources which cannot be cast aside. For example, the Inter-Society Commission for Heart Disease Resources reported in 1970 that a narrowing of arteries by atherosclerosis cannot occur in animals experimentally without a drastic change in the animal's diet. The diet change consists of increasing the proportion of cholesterol and fat, which in turn increases the levels of these substances in the animal's bloodstream.

The International Cooperative Study on the Epidemiology of Cardiovascular Disease presents dietary data on human beings. Twelve thousand men, originally in the 40 to 59 age group, were studied in seven countries—Finland, the United States, Greece, Italy, Japan, the Netherlands, and Yugoslavia. The men in the study were followed for ten years. A wide difference was found in the prevalence of coronary heart disease—heart attacks—between the seven countries. Eastern Finland had six times and the United States four times the incidence of heart attacks as was found in certain Greek Islands and Japan. An analysis of the diets among men from the different countries revealed that in the Japanese diet, total fat represented only nine percent of calories consumed, while in the Netherlands and the United States, total fat represented from 35 to 40 percent of calories ingested. The fat intake in eastern Finland was even higher.

Many other studies could be quoted, including autopsy studies from different countries, which all point in the same direction. People who consume greater amounts of fats and cholesterol in their diets develop more heart attacks and consequently have a shorter life span than people living on lower fat diets. The fats and cholesterol in the diet are carried into the bloodstream where they invade the inner lining of the arteries. The result is the development of patches of arteriosclerosis, and this development starts very early in life.

From this discussion it is obvious that we are going to have to regulate the quantity of fat and cholesterol in our diets if we are going to protect ourselves from the coronary epidemic.

Cholesterol. What is a "safe" level of cholesterol and where do we find cholesterol in our food? Cholesterol is present in our blood as one of the normal body fats, and the quantity present in each individual can be determined by a simple blood test. Some people have the mistaken idea that cholesterol is a foreign substance in the body. Doctors often have the question asked of them, "Do I have any cholesterol, Doc?" The point of concern is not whether we have any, but rather, do we have too much.

The answer to the question "Is my cholesterol too high?" appears to be that the less cholesterol present in your blood, the better off you are. Literature from the public health agencies will often state that cholesterol levels less than 200 are normal, those between 200 and 249 are borderline, and levels above 250 are abnormal for adults over the age of thirty. These figures are really only guidelines. The reason that these particular levels were chosen is because those persons who have a cholesterol level over 250 have twice the risk of developing premature coronary heart disease as those persons who have a level below this figure. However, the person who has a cholesterol level of 210 has a greater risk than the person with a level of 160. Moderately elevated cholesterol also becomes much more significant in the individual who also has other factors substantially affecting his chances of having a heart attack—factors such as cigarette smoking and high blood pressure.

As far as our knowledge goes today, there is no known disease associated solely with low blood cholesterol. In other words, the fortunate person who may have a cholesterol of 100 is not destined to develop any form of health deficiency due to the low cholesterol level. The logical approach, therefore, appears to be for each person to strive for as low a level of cholesterol as possible without, of course, centering their entire life's purpose around this one factor.

Ten years ago most physicians were rather fatalistic about changing the course of atherosclerosis or hardening of the arteries in man. It was felt that changes in the diet might help to prevent the further development of atherosclerosis, but that the damage already done would undoubtedly persist.

However, experiments on simple animal forms revealed that the change from a high to a low cholesterol diet would result in the disappearance of patches of atherosclerosis that had been formed, and later experiments on primates (monkeys) confirmed these findings. Now Dr. Jeremiah Stamler, Chairman of the Department of Community Health and Preventive Medicine at the Northwestern University Medical School, states that reports indicate that a reduction in the calorie, fat, and cholesterol intake can lead to a reduction in the size of patches of atherosclerosis in *man*. With this encouraging information, let's delve into our diet to see what modifications may be necessary to lower our cholesterol.

The main source of cholesterol in the average American diet is egg yolks. About 35 percent of our total cholesterol intake comes from this single item. Meat, poultry, fish, and shellfish combine to contribute another 35 percent, and dairy products add about 15 percent. As a matter of comparison, one egg yolk contains about 300 mg of cholesterol while an ounce of meat contains about 30 mg. The average American consumes about 1000 mg of cholesterol a day. Foods with a significant cholesterol content are egg yolks; shellfish, including lobster, oysters, scallops, clams, shrimp, and crab; organ meats, such as liver, brains, heart, kidneys, sweetbreads, and fish roe, including caviar; dairy products containing fat, such as whole milk, butter, cream (sweet or sour), ice cream, hard cheese, cream cheese, and creamed cottage cheese; and animal fat.

The body also has the capacity to produce cholesterol. The principal raw materials used for this purpose are saturated fats. The fats in our diet can be separated roughly into those which are saturated and those which are unsaturated. The difference is determined by the chemical structure of the fat. Fats of animal origin are saturated; vegetable fats are primarily unsaturated unless treated chemically (by the addition of hydrogen) to be converted into a solid form. In other words, hard cooking shortening is saturated, whereas the liquid cooking oils are unsaturated. There is even a difference among the liquids. Those cooking oils and margarines made from either safflower or corn oil are more unsaturated than those made from olive oil and peanut oil. Coconut oil is an exception; although it is of vegetable origin, it is a saturated fat.

It now becomes apparent that, in addition to watching out for foods which have a high cholesterol content (see the preceding list), we have to be conservative with foods which contain saturated fat. Foods with a significant content of saturated fats are animal fat, such as lard, suet, salt pork, and bacon and meat drippings; meats with a high fat content, such as regular hamburger, hot dogs, luncheon meat, sausage, bacon, spare ribs, marbled steaks, all fatty meats, goose, duck, and poultry skin; spreads and oils such as butter, hydrogenated margarine and shortening, coconut oil (substitute safflower oil, corn oil, soft safflower margarine, or commercial mayonnaise); commercial baked goods made with lard or hydrogenated shortening; and frozen or packaged products with the above contents.

If a serious cholesterol problem is present, it may also be necessary to reduce the quantity of beef, lamb, ham, and pork in the diet. This is due to the fat contained in these meats which cannot be removed by trimming prior to or after cooking. A strict reduction might be down to a level of three servings of three ounces per week. Fish and poultry (without the skin) are lower in fat than other forms of meat and should be used as a substitute for meat whenever possible.

The first thought which comes to many persons on reading over this list of foods is that there are very few things that they enjoy which are not prohibited. This is true for most Americans because the classic diet is ham and eggs, hot dogs or hamburgers, and marbled steaks with a baked potato drowned in butter and sour cream. The truth remains, however, that a change must be made. The easiest place to start is by searching for painless substitutions. The use of corn or safflower oils and margarines for lard, solid shortening, and butter is an example. This shift should be possible without the ruffling of too many feathers.

Since egg yolks are so high in cholesterol, a very effective way to decrease the cholesterol intake is to make the usual breakfast of eggs and bacon or sausage a Sunday treat instead of an everyday affair. An acceptable substitute would be dry or cooked cereal and various types of breads supplemented with fruits and juices. If a hard-working man requires more calories in the mornings, a piece of broiled fish or lean meat would be far better for him than eggs and pork.

At what age should a person start to concern himself with the level of cholesterol in his blood? Scientists have not arrived at a uniform recommendation on this subject. However, the earlier in life that attention is paid to the prevention of heart attacks, the more successful the results will be. It would appear logical for persons in the 25- to 30-year-old age bracket to find out where they stand.

In certain cases, particularly those in which extremely high cholesterol levels are found or in which the blood cholesterol levels do not respond adequately to diet, physicians may prescribe some form of drug treatment. One of the most promising drugs in this category is clofibrate (Atromid-S®). Approximately 65 percent of those men with an elevated cholesterol level treated with clofibrate responded with a reduction in their cholesterol on the order of from 15 to 20 percent.

Drs. Krasno and Kidera of the Clinical Research Division of United Air Lines ran a study of over 3,000 men for a period of time (from 22 to 39 months) and determined that men given clofibrate had a significantly decreased incidence of heart attacks compared to a like group of men who had not taken the drug.

Work of this nature offers hope for those persons who have not been able to control their cholesterol by diet, particularly if they are members of a high risk category, such as victims of a previous heart attack or those with a high incidence of heart attacks in older family members.

Triglycerides. These are another class of fats found normally in our bloodstreams. If abnormally high levels are present, they contribute to the formation of patches of arteriosclerosis in the arteries of our bodies.

Trigylcerides are a component of various types of the fats we eat. They find their way into our circulation after digestion and absorption have taken place in our intestines. A certain proportion of trigylcerides is produced within the body. The raw materials for their production are carbohydrates (starches and sugars) and alcohol.

The blood test for cholesterol remains the best single blood examination that can be used for estimating the risk of premature coronary heart disease. If the cholesterol test results are unusually high, the physician will often test for triglycerides also. There are certain conditions which run in families (rather rare) in which one or both of these tests are abnormal. High blood fats may also appear as a secondary feature in certain diseases of the thyroid gland, liver, kidneys, or pancreas and in diabetes and alcoholism. If a physician suspects any of these conditions, additional testing is required.

High Calorie Diets. Our rich modern diet is directly responsible for the fact that 20 percent of the teen-agers and 50 percent of the middle-aged adults in our country are overweight (obese). This obesity represents a significant risk factor in the development of premature coronary heart disease because overweight individuals are more likely to develop hypertension and diabetes. People with these latter two diseases carry a much greater risk of developing a coronary heart disease and heart attack because they develop atherosclerosis in their arteries at an accelerated pace.

Why does a person become overweight? The answer is not complicated. The heavy person has consumed more calories in food than he has burned up by physical activity over a period of time. Despite hundreds of books which have been written on the subject, the answer is that simple in 99 percent of overweight people.

An interesting study was just conducted by Dr. Ralph Nelson of the Mayo Clinic. The study attempted to find the answer to why obese persons are overweight. They attempted to answer three assumptions that have been made about this problem. First, obese persons are overweight because they use calories more economically than normal weight persons (they have a lower "metabolism"). The second proposition maintains that obese persons have difficulty in using up their body fat for energy needs. The third assumption tested was that the obese are heavy because they eat more than people who are normal weight.

Dr. Nelson and his group studied 142 persons including normal weight adults, obese adults, normal weight and obese adolescents. The results of their studies contradict some long held myths about obesity. First of all, the obese used carbohydrates, fats, and proteins normally during rest and exercise and did not have a different "metabolism." Furthermore, the obese used fat deposits for the production of energy more readily than normal persons did. Finally, some "normal" persons became obese with age without changing their eating and exercise habits. The key to the problem here is that the metabolism of the body decreases with advancing age, and even if most persons decrease the amount of food which they eat, they will become fat if they maintain the same level of exercise. Put in other terms, the body becomes more efficient with age, and less food is required to maintain a normal weight. The only way that a person in his forties or fifties can maintain an ideal weight is to dramatically reduce his total calorie intake or significantly increase the amount of calories that he burns through exercise. This change begins when a person is in his thirties, so adjustments must be made at this early age to prevent the development of obesity.

These findings substantiate the feelings of many overweight middle-aged persons who protest to their doctors that they are mysteriously gaining weight despite the fact that they are eating much less than they used to. It is also a fairly universal fact that people tend to be less active physically as they grow older. These two factors, a decreased amount of activity and a decreased need by the body for food, are responsible for the nagging weight gain which plagues many Americans who are beyond their mid-thirties.

Is there any easy answer to the problem? Yes, as long as you start the solution to your problem with the above facts. If you are gaining weight, or if you are unable to lose weight, you must either cut down on the average daily intake of calories, or you must increase the amount of food that you burn up through physical activity, or both.

At this point in such a discussion, a patient will often state, "I don't understand what calories are, I count carbohydrates instead. And even though I count my carbohydrates, I'm still gaining weight." This brings us back to the basic plan behind diets. A few words of explanation may clear up a great deal of misunderstanding. We've already said that 50 percent of the middle-aged adults in this country are overweight, so obviously we're dealing with a problem that affects a fantastic number of persons. In response to this problem, many people have tried to devise diets that are comfortable to follow—diets which appeal to different types of people. The egg diet, wine diet, grapefruit diet, carbohydrate diet, and of course, the Air Force diet, are examples. The basic objective of all of these diets is weight loss. The only difference is in the method proposed. Because different things appeal to different people and because individuals have a varied level of understanding, shortcuts have been devised. The basic ingredient of all of these diets has been an attempt to decrease the amount of foods, and particularly of high caloric foods, which people eat. Some diets become distasteful, so they accomplish their goal through the loss of appetite. An excellent example of this is the high fat diet.

This is the reason that drugs are sometimes prescribed to curb the appetite. Of interest is the fact that recent investigations have led the Federal Food and Drug Administration to advise physicians that these drugs usually have the desired effect for only a relatively short period of time. The fact that many people are unable to lose weight with these medicines attests to the fact that they have a limited usefulness.

Much of this activity has developed because people have a fear of the unknown when it comes to "counting calories." The average person doesn't understand what calories are and gets confused trying to count them. The same confusion would exist if we measured gasoline in America in liters, as they do in Europe, instead of in gallons. If the change were imposed by government order however, most of us would soon learn that a liter is almost equivalent to a quart and that four liters is just a little bit more than a gallon.

A calorie is no more than a simple measurement of the energy which different foods contain. As far as food economics is concerned, we have to appreciate that most foods contain calories, some more than others. If we only concern ourselves with counting carbohydrates, for example, we are ignoring the energy that we eat in the form of protein (meat) and fats (butter and cream). All three of the basic foods, carbohydrates, fats, and proteins, contain calories. Therefore, we have to be concerned with all the foods we eat (and with the liquids we drink). If you are unable to lose weight and are eating a 2500 calorie diet each day, the logical thing to do is to reduce the food intake to 2000 calories a day. If a weight loss still doesn't occur, reduce it further.

The alternative is to increase your physical activity so that you are burning up more calories than usual. The goal is to achieve a balance between the calories that you eat and those which you spend through activity. If you are burning up more than you consume, you will eventually lose weight. If you are consuming more than you burn up through activity, you will gain weight. You don't have to be a scientist or a mathematician to figure out how many calories you are using each day; your scales will tell you the answer.

Many people get into trouble in the area of prepared foods. How many calories does a chicken pot pie have? How many calories were in the hamburger that you had for lunch? What does this particular doughnut contain? Realizing the importance of this problem, the government is starting to require food-packaging companies to list the calorie content of prepared foods. Hopefully, in the near future, all canned and packaged foods will have an accurate labeling of the calorie and nutritional content of each product.

The final area of difficulty lies in being sure that a person is obtaining all of the essential foods that are necessary for health during a period of dieting. Recent studies have shown that large segments of our population are actually undernourished, despite the fact that they consume adequate amounts of food.

There is a very simple way to get factual advice on this matter. If you are unable to lose weight, or if you are in doubt about the nutritional content of your diet, make a list of all the foods you eat in the space of a week. Include everything, especially drinks (including alcoholic beverages) and snacks. Take the list to your physician, and he will help you to evaluate your diet. If he is unable to provide this service, he will refer you to a dietician at your local hospital where you can usually get good advice at a reasonable charge.

In addition to calculating the calories which you are consuming, professional advice can often help you to decide on the forms of physical activity which you can participate in to increase the number of calories you burn each day.

Hypertension—High Blood Pressure. High blood pressure, along with elevated blood cholesterol and cigarette smoking, is one of the most important risk factors in the development of premature coronary heart disease.

Hypertension stands alone as a risk factor and has increased importance if a person has one or two of the other risk factors as well. Based on studies of population samples, it is estimated that 20 million Americans have high blood pressure and that at least half of this number have no idea they have the disease. The reason for this is that hypertension does not produce symptoms until the elevated pressure reaches very high levels or until complications of the disease have occurred—complications such as a heart attack, stroke, or heart failure. A person may harbor hypertension for from two to ten or more years before any symptoms or complications force the discovery of the problem. This points up the fact that Americans must get into the habit of having their blood pressures checked periodically.

Dr. G. E. Burch of the Tulane University School of Medicine feels so strongly about the problem of undetected hypertension that he has proposed that every home in America have a device to periodically measure blood pressure, just as every home should be equipped with a thermometer. This suggestion may not be economically practical, but as a rule of thumb, persons in their twenties and thirties should have their blood pressure checked at least once a year, and persons over that age should have it tested two or three times annually.

Studies have also suggested that only from 25 to 30 percent of the people who know that they have high blood pressure are adequately treated for the problem. There are many reasons for this, to be sure, but one of the most important reasons is that the affected person often feels well and doesn't appreciate the consequences of uncontrolled hypertension. Persons whose diastolic blood pressure is 105 or greater have three times as many heart attacks as those with a diastolic blood pressure below 85. Fortunately, excellent drugs are available that can control almost all cases of hypertension.

What is a normal blood pressure? Apparently just as in the case of cholesterol, the lower the blood pressure (within reason), the lower the risk of eventually provoking a heart attack. This answer avoids the question for most readers, so in general, for a middle-aged person, a blood pressure below 140/90 is "normal." Certainly a blood pressure over 160/95 would warrant treatment of some sort. A person in his fifties.or sixties might be considered normal if his pressure was below 150/90.

For further discussion of hypertension, the reader is referred to the separate chapter in this book which covers the topic in more detail.

Cigarette Smoking. The third important factor that predisposes Americans to a high risk of premature death from heart attack, besides hypertension and a high calorie, high fat, and high cholesterol diet, is cigarette smoking.

Convincing people that cigarette smoking is dangerous is difficult. Despite the fact that the government has been able to force tobacco manufacturers to label cigarette packages with the warning that "Smoking Is Dangerous to Your Health" and despite the fact that they have been able to force cigarette commercials off the television channels, people continue to smoke in large numbers. The cigarette habit is obviously one that has a deep emotional and psychological hold on a great deal of our fellow Americans, so we won't counter their habit with a sermon. Instead, let's deal with facts.

Fact one: men and women in a developed country who smoke over a pack of cigarettes a day have three times the risk of having a heart attack that a non-smoker has.

Fact two: the younger the person and the greater the cigarette consumption, the greater the risk of heart attack.

Fact three: women who are heavy cigarette smokers are as susceptible to death from heart attacks as men.

Let's examine these facts further. In the first statement, we used the qualifying statement, "in a developed country." These statistics are most significant in countries where a high cholesterol, high fat, and high calorie diet are associated with a prevalence of other factors predisposing to premature coronary heart disease.

It appears that cigarette smoking by itself may not aggravate the development of "hardening" of the arteries (arteriosclerosis), but if arteriosclerosis is already present, cigarette smoking somehow increases the risk of a heart attack and particularly the risk of sudden death from a heart attack.

It is interesting that most Americans associate cigarette smoking with a greater chance of developing cancer of the lung or emphysema. Actually, their fears are misdirected. All types of cancer, including cancer of the lung, breast, uterus, stomach, colon, kidney, and brain, account for less than half the number of deaths in the United States that heart attacks cause. The biggest danger of cigarette smoking is death from a heart attack.

Women are generally considered to be protected to a great extent against heart attacks until after the menopause. Statistics tell us that men have five times as many heart attacks as women before the menopausal age. After this period of life, women gradually catch up to men as far as the incidence of heart attacks is concerned.

A recent study of autopsy data collected by Dr. David Spain of Brooklyn reveals that, though twenty years ago men under 51 years of age were 12 times more vulnerable than women to sudden death from heart attacks, data collected between 1967 and 1971 reveal that this ratio has changed to four to one. The difference in this death rate is attributed by Dr. Spain to the increase in heavy cigarette smoking in women.

It is interesting that persons who smoke cigars or pipes have no greater chance of having a heart attack than non-smokers. It is also interesting that the smoker who gives up the habit rapidly reduces his risk of heart attack to nearly as low a level as the habitual non-smoker. Furthermore, a pack a day or more man is exposing himself to twice the risk of a person who smokes less than half a pack per day.

Enough for statistics. What mechanism is responsible for cigarettes causing these heart problems? We're not sure, but it is known that nicotine increases the heart rate and also increases the tendency of blood to clot.

Investigations have turned up a new twist that has broad implications in our way of life. Carbon monoxide has become a prime suspect as the mechanism for cigarette-induced sudden heart death. Cigarette smoking, as well as automobile engines and indoor fires used for the production of house warming, all produce carbon monoxide as a by-product of the combustion (burning) of "fuel" (whether it be tobacco, gasoline, or charcoal).

Carbon monoxide is an invisible gas that mixes easily with air and is breathed into our lungs. Once inside the body, carbon monoxide is treated as if it were royalty. For unknown reasons, our red blood cells (which are responsible for carrying oxygen to all parts of our bodies) treat carbon monoxide in a preferential manner. The hemoglobin in the red blood cell, which is the chemical that carries oxygen, is 300 times more ready to carry carbon monoxide than it is to carry oxygen. The result is that when a person breathes even small amounts of carbon monoxide (such as that contained in a cigarette) his red blood cells are going to be carrying much less oxygen than normal. Since a heart attack is due to a blood vessel (which supplies the heart with oxygen) becoming blocked, it is easy to see how cigarettes can increase the risk of heart death.

A forty-year-old man has narrowing of his coronary arteries by arteriosclerosis, but he has never had symptoms from the disease—it hasn't progressed far enough. On a particular day he is tense and anxious over a business deal. He smokes an unusual number of cigarettes. The carbon monoxide in the cigarettes combines preferentially with the hemoglobin in his red blood cells, and the blood is able to carry less and less oxygen to his heart. His anxiety is stimulating his glands to produce more adrenaline. His heart beats faster and therefore requires more oxygen for nourishment. A certain critical point is reached, and the heart revolts against the abnormally low oxygen supply. The nervous system of the heart goes into rebellion, and the result is a total disorganization of the heartbeat—known medically as ventricular fibrillation. Within five minutes the victim is dead.

There really is no alternative. If we want to survive the coronary epidemic, we are going to have to rearrange our smoking habits. The options in decreasing order of preference are: to stop smoking cigarettes altogether, to smoke only cigars or a pipe, or to smoke less than half a pack of cigarettes a day. The latter suggestion shouldn't be too difficult for even the veteran smoker to accept.

Physical Inactivity. Most experts agree that the main factors with which we have to concern ourselves in preventing heart attacks are obesity, a high cholesterol level, cigarette smoking, and hypertension. There are other factors which are considered significant, although possibly not as important as these three. A lack of regular physical exercise is in this latter category. The reason that it is considered to be a minor factor is in part due to the difficulty in accumulating hard evidence to support the concept. This may be due to the fact that it is a minor factor, or it may be due to the fact that we are not capable of dissecting all the factors in our lives which are resulting in our being victims of the coronary epidemic. In other words, we may be in the position of the horse or dog. The animal realizes that he feels better when he drinks water; he is no longer thirsty. However, the animal doesn't have the scientific knowledge to understand either that he requires drinking water to replace the water lost by his body through the processes of perspiration and urination or that, if he doesn't drink water, he will eventually die from dehydration.

There are a number of studies which have been performed on groups of people in an attempt to clarify the problem We will examine only one of them to understand why many investigators of heart disease believe that regular exercise may have a very important part to play in preventing heart attacks.

In 1960, Dr. Curtis Hames of Evans County, Georgia,

enlisted the aid of the Department of Epidemiology at the University of North Carolina to help him to establish the reasons for an observation that he had made during his years of practice in the area. He was impressed by the fact that black men whom he treated rarely had heart attacks, despite the fact that these same men frequently had significant hypertension. The matter was more intriguing because Evans County happens to be in an area of the Southeast where deaths from heart attacks are common in white patients and are occurring more frequently than in many other parts of the United States. Accordingly, every resident of the county over the age of forty and 50 percent of the population between the ages of fifteen and thirty-nine were examined and given laboratory tests by two doctors over the next year and a half. The 3,102 persons examined represented 92 percent of all those persons in the above age groups. The same group of individuals were reexamined between 1967 and 1969.

Analysis of the data from these studies confirmed Dr. Hames' impressions. Black men had less than half the number of heart attacks that white men had endured. Attempting to find the reason for this difference, the standard risk factors were analyzed—blood pressure, cholesterol, cigarette smoking, diet, and body weight. There were no significant differences in the presence of these risk factors that could divine a reason for the low heart attack rate in black men.

Further analysis of the data revealed the striking fact that one social class of white men had as low an incidence of heart attacks as black men had. These men were sharecroppers. There were no significant differences in the weight, smoking habits, cholesterol, or blood pressure between the white sharecroppers and other white men. The only factor that appeared to be a common denominator between the white sharecroppers and the black men was a high level of physical activity. The results of this unique study cannot be transposed to the entire United States, but certainly in Evans County, Georgia, the extreme physical activity that is involved in farming (if one is the working farm hand) seems to protect one against heart attacks.

By what means could exercise protect us against heart attacks? The answer to this question is also unknown. We do know that the heart of an athlete is more efficient than that of the average person. The heart beats slower at rest and at work and seems to pump blood with less effort. In addition, exercise lowers various types of fats in the blood stream, which may decrease the likelihood that these fats will filter out into the lining of the blood vessels and cause atherosclerotic obstructions. People who exercise regularly also appear to be able to carry more oxygen in their blood, and they may have a decreased tendency to form blood clots. There is no specific answer, but circumstantial evidence is very strong in suggesting that exercise may help our hearts a great deal.

The next logical question is—what type of exercise can I do? This will depend on your age and the extent of your present physical conditioning. Regardless of your age, it is usually not advisable to suddenly change from a life of gross inactivity to that of a superathlete. You should work up gradually into new forms of strenuous activity. And if you happen to be over the age of thirty-five or forty, you would be wise to have a physical examination before you start an exercise program. Have your physician give you specific advice on how rapidly you should proceed into strenuous activity. If you are not in good physical condition, and particularly if you have some type of heart disease or do not feel as well as you think you should, it is imperative that you check with your doctor before you start any form of increased exercise. Otherwise, you could push yourself into some type of serious heart malfunction.

One of the ways that your doctor can help guide you in an exercise program is by testing your response to simple exercise in his office. There are tables which suggest the maximum increase in the heart rate which persons should allow themselves to attain at different age levels. For example, a person in the forty- to forty-nine-year age group should not push himself in exercise beyond that point which would cause an acceleration of his pulse beyond 140 or 145 beats per minute. The very important exception to this is if the person being tested develops symptoms such as unusual tiredness, shortness of breath, rapid heartbeat, or any degree of chest discomfort. Many doctors will have a patient exercise in their office, doing stationary jogging or other forms of activity, and will then examine the person on the spot to see what effect this level of exercise produces on their heart action, pulse, and blood pressure. In some cases electrocardiograms are taken during or immediately after exercise to assist an evaluation. The doctor may even teach the person how to take his pulse rate and instruct him to check his pulse after a period of exercise. If the pulse is exceeding certain limits, a decrease in the intensity of exercise is necessary.

The Inter-Society Commission for Heart Disease Resources reported in 1970 the following regarding exercise:

> Regular exercise, particularly those forms of endurance exercise which enhance cardiovascular fitness, may have a role to play in the prevention of atherosclerotic diseases. It is im-

portant to emphasize, however, that exercise is not free of danger both to the musculoskeletal system and the cardiovascular systems. This is particularly true for middle-aged individuals—especially coronary-prone persons—who suddenly take up vigorous exercise after years of minimal physical activity. Physicians and other professionals need aid in guiding a concerned public to avoid these problems. Research on the role and programming of exercise for the prevention of atherosclerotic diseases must be pursued vigorously to obtain more definitive information.

Certainly, if a person has any form of heart disease, he should definitely consult his physician about the level of physical exercise which he can safely pursue. There is good evidence to believe that physical exercise will benefit these persons as well as those who have never had any evidence of heart trouble.

Drs. Samuel Fox, John Naughton, and Patrick Gorman of the George Washington School of Medicine recently discussed physical activity in *Modern Concepts of Cardiovascular Disease,* a publication of the American Heart Association. The following chart represents a résumé of the relative demands various forms of activity place on the body.

Class of Activity	Typical Occupation	Typical Recreational Activity
1	Desk work or driving a car	Standing, walking one mile/hr, playing cards, sewing, or knitting
2	Auto repair, radio, TV repair, janitorial work, or bartending	Level walking 2 mile/hr, level bicycling 5 miles/hr, shuffleboard, operating a powerboat, golf with a power cart, or playing piano and many other musical instruments

Class of Activity	Typical Occupation	Typical Recreational Activity
3	Bricklaying, plastering, wheelbarrow 100 lb. load, machine assembly, welding, trailer-truck in traffic, or cleaning windows	Walking 3 miles/hr, bicycling 6 miles/hr, pitching horseshoes, golf pulling bag cart, sailing small boat, horseback riding to trot, badminton doubles, or pushing light power mower
4	Painting, paperhanging, or light carpentry	Walking 3½ miles/hr, bicycling 8 miles/hr, table tennis, dancing foxtrot, badminton singles, tennis doubles, raking leaves, or many calisthenics
5	Digging garden or shoveling light earth	Canoeing 4 miles/hr, horseback riding ("posting" to trot), or ice or roller skating 9 miles/hr
6	Shoveling 10 lbs 10 times a minute	Walking 5 miles/hr, bicycling 11 miles/hr, tennis singles, splitting wood, snow shoveling, hand lawn-mowing, folk dancing, light downhill skiing, or water skiing
7	Digging ditches, carrying 80 lbs, or sawing hardwood	Jogging 5 miles/hr, bicycling 12 miles/hr, horseback (gallop), vigorous downhill skiing, basketball, mountain climbing, ice hockey, or touch football
8	Shoveling 14 lbs 10 times a minute	Running 5½ miles/hr, bicycling 13 miles/hr, ski touring 4 miles/hr (loose snow), handball or squash (social), fencing, or basketball (vigorous)

Since people perform these types of activity with different intensity, whether a person approaches the matter with a frenzy or with a casual attitude will make a big difference in the amount of energy spent. Therefore, the calculation of a person's pulse rate in the middle of a particular exercise is still a better gauge of how the body is reacting to the exercise.

Frantic Pace of Life. Our life style, or pace, undoubtedly plays a role in determining whether or not we will develop premature coronary heart disease. This is the most difficult of all factors to analyze and therefore to offer concrete recommendations about. It is considered an important element because of facts which do not appear to be coincidental. The usual coronary risk factors are significant in a modern industrialized society, but they carry much less weight when examined in casual, pastoral societies.

Dr. Meyer Friedman at the Mount Zion Hospital in San Francisco and his co-workers have studied this factor in depth. They have come to the conclusion that they are able to identify the person who is most likely to develop a coronary, and the identification is based solely on personality traits. Dr. Friedman calls this susceptible personality a Type A individual. According to his studies, the Type A person is two and a half times more likely to have a heart attack than a Type B person. In people under the age of fifty, the ratio rises to three to one.

The Type A person is competitive and aggressive. He is constantly driving and extremely time conscious. This person is very punctual and resents being held up for any reason, whether it be in a traffic jam, waiting for service in a restaurant, or for appointments. He is always on time and is very intolerant of any person who keeps him waiting. He is constantly striving to utilize every moment because he never has enough time to do all of the things which he considers necessary. He is constantly striving for new goals and belittling his past accomplishments. During ordinary conversation, it is often easy to pick out the Type A. He will often interrupt the person who is talking to finish the sentence.

Another characteristic is polyphasic thinking. This means that he is thinking of two or more things at the same time. He is listening to a conversation and dwelling over another matter. These people read while they eat. Attention to routine tasks is difficult or impossible, because he is thinking of one thing while he does another. This characteristic is responsible for one of his true weaknesses: he often accomplishes things rapidly, but tasks are often not well done. He may be successful in his work, but it is despite this fault. A Type B person is more deliberate, spends more time analyzing the situation before acting, and therefore makes less mistakes. A very successful person may as well be a Type B as a Type A. The Type A is found in all walks of life—from truck drivers and mechanics to businessmen. The person in the lower economic category will often have a second job to fully use his productive time.

The Type A is very competitive. He is much less likely to be interested in gardening than in golf or tennis, where he can bet and compete against fellow players. His sense of insecurity makes him strive and compete constantly, so that in his relations with other people, he is always trying to outdo or belittle them.

Another characteristic is an obsession with numbers. Dollars in the bank, number of clients served in one day, the total sales for the week: these are the tools with which he gauges the success or failure of his material day. His values are in having things rather than in being someone or in enjoying art, literature, or nature.

The Type A places very little value on love, friendship, and emotion. He rarely takes vacations, and when he does, it is not usually to relax. He is more apt to combine some form of business with a vacation or to compete, such as in hunting or fishing, against other people.

Dr. Friedman believes that the Type A individual will succumb to a heart attack regardless of what he does to alter his weight, cholesterol, blood pressure, or smoking habits. How could this type of drive affect the body to produce a heart attack? It probably has something to do with chemicals that are released into the body during stress. Scientific measurements have shown that during stress adrenaline concentrations increase in the blood and elevations occur in the cholesterol content of the blood. At autopsy, these men all have significant coronary artery disease. Their predisposition to heart attacks could be due to adrenaline stimulating the nervous system control of the heart to start up irregular heartbeats and particularly fibrillations. Hearts with narrowed coronary arteries are very susceptible to erratic behavior when these chemicals are present in high concentrations in the bloodstream.

If this description of the Type A personality fits you, you would be very smart to attempt to change your behavior. The job will be difficult, but it can be done. Dr. Friedman was a Type A himself before he had his heart attack. He has trained himself to be a Type B. His suggestions for accomplishing this are as follows:

Stop polyphasic thinking. Whenever you catch yourself thinking about two things at the same time—stop. This is a significant symptom that must be curbed.

Stop watching the clock and counting numbers. Analyze this behavior. Consider what you are doing in terms of how important it will be one or five years from now. Will you lose your job if you're five minutes late for work—or should the waitress lose hers? Does it really make a difference to have an extra 500 dollars in the bank when you retire?

Stop interrupting people. Let your wife talk for a change and listen to what she has to say. You could find it interesting after a while, in the enjoyment that she receives from having you listen if not in the content of what she is saying.

Learn to enjoy food. Many Type A persons never really taste the food they eat or the beverages they drink. Don't use mealtimes for a place to do battle or conduct business. Share interesting experiences with partners.

Avoid irritating people and nonessential activities as far as possible, except of course, for those absolutely necessary for business. Meetings that you hate to attend and people who irritate and bring out your aggressive nature should be dropped like poison.

Take some time out of every day to enjoy yourself and life; plan trips and vacations that are relaxing. A part of each day should be spent by yourself relaxing and thinking. Take a walk through a park, stroll through a museum, drive leisurely through a scenic part of town on your way to work, and pay attention to the scenery. Wake up early enough in the morning to dress and breakfast leisurely. Take a long lunch that is not tied in with business.

Avoid business trips in which you travel to a distant city, have meetings, and return the same day. Take an extra day or two to rest either coming or going, and combine some form of pleasant activity with the work day.

Finally, vacations should be planned so that there is no

association with work or competition in any way. A vacation should be a time to forget about business worries and to recharge your batteries through different, relaxed, pleasant activities. If these are spent with a mate or children, take the time to enjoy them, learn to understand and love them for what they are.

All the things that we have discussed in this chapter, diet, general physical health, exercise, and a relaxed mental outlook, will probably contribute a great deal to avoiding a premature heart attack. These same things will also result in your improving the quality of the life you are living. The person who is at his ideal weight feels better inside because he knows that he looks better than his obese neighbor. The person who regularly exercises in some fashion that is enjoyable to him feels better because he is more relaxed and has less aches and pains from idleness. The Type A individual who has changed his ways feels better because he's taking the time to see how he feels and to enjoy all the life that surrounds him.

After all, I'm sure that we would all agree that we are more interested in a quality life—a life that is full of interest, warmth, love, and pure enjoyment—than a long life that is tedious and boring. Wake up all you Type A people! Start to really enjoy each day that you're living, or one day you may have only a sorrowful, though rich, widow to grieve your passing.

19

Emergency Check List

Over 2,000,000 Americans will have heart attacks this year, and about 700,000 of these will die. Probably half of those who die from a heart attack will never reach a hospital. The primary reason for this is that most people are not aware that they are having a heart attack. The best way that we can save more lives is to awaken those people who may be in trouble to the fact that they should seek help quickly. The following list of symptoms is provided as a guideline to help you to decide whether or not you are having heart symptoms. If there is any doubt at all in your mind, don't hesitate any further, call your doctor or go to your nearest emergency room and get direct advice.

When you call your doctor, don't be hesitant or embarrassed. Tell him directly that you're afraid that you are having either a heart attack or some other form of heart trouble. Many times a person will have a sixth sense that he is having a heart attack—if you feel this, say so. This is especially important if you are going to a crowded emergency room. Announce your presence to the receptionist and say that you think you're having a heart attack. The place for you at that time is with a doctor and not in a crowded room waiting for your turn to come up.

Chest Pain. A heart attack usually produces discomfort in the chest. Some people describe the discomfort as a pain, others use terms such as a pressure, tightness, or constriction, usually located behind the breastbone or sternum, in the center of the chest. The pain may also be felt in the neck, jaw, shoulders, or arms. At times the discomfort seems to travel through to the back. If a person is having a heart attack, the pain persists for half an hour, an hour, or longer. The pain is not fleeting—lasting for just a few seconds and then disappearing.

About a third of the people having a heart attack will have experienced the same pain in a milder form, often lasting for only one, two, or five minutes and reoccurring over a few days or a few weeks before the actual heart attack. These have been warning pains that should have taken the person to medical attention.

One of the most important features about this chest discomfort is that it is a new experience. It is usually not the type of thing that you have been feeling off and on for years. The fact that this is a new pain occurring in the front of the chest is enough reason to suspect a heart attack. Contact your doctor immediately or go to the nearest emergency room and report your symptoms. Don't be afraid to tell the doctor or nurse that you think you're having a heart attack.

Indigestion. Probably half of the people having a heart attack call it indigestion. They often describe the feeling as a fullness or weight in the pit of the stomach or in the very lower part of the chest. They usually take some form of an antacid (often a seltzer), belch, and feel better for a few moments before the discomfort returns. The fact that you can belch and feel better for a moment does not prove that this is indigestion. Heart attacks often occur after big meals. If the discomfort is not completely relieved by a simple home measure, or if it is a new type of indigestion, call your doctor or go to the nearest emergency room. You may be having a heart attack. Say so.

Sweating, Nausea, Vomiting. These symptoms may accompany a heart attack, and they are therefore not an indication that you are merely dealing with indigestion. These symptoms do not always accompany a heart attack, however, and therefore if you don't have them, it doesn't mean that you are not having a heart attack.

Fainting. A person with a severe heart attack may lose consciousness and fall to the ground. This is a very serious sign as it usually means that the heart is not pumping blood and that immediate resuscitation may be necessary. Fainting does not always accompany a heart attack. If you are having chest discomfort and do not faint, this does not mean that your trouble is not your heart. Many people mistakenly believe that all heart attacks are associated with pain, sweating, shortness of breath, and fainting. This is not true. Only some heart attacks have all of these symptoms.

Any adult person who faints should seek immediate medical attention unless he has a seizure disorder (such as epilepsy) or has been fainting for some time from minor shocks, such as pain or the sight of blood. The usual reason for an adult fainting is that his heart is not pumping blood to his brain, and whether this is due to a heart attack or to some other form of heart or brain disorder, it requires immediate attention. If you faint, call your doctor or go to the nearest emergency room.

Lapses, Slipping Away, Floating, Fluttering Chest. During a heart attack, sometimes the heart does not beat correctly. There may be a series of rapid, faint beats followed by a regular beat or there may be a continuous very rapid heartbeat. In both these cases, patients may not actually faint, but the pumping action of the heart may be below normal. Although the brain is receiving enough blood to prevent a loss of consciousness, it is not receiving enough oxygen to prevent some degree of malfunction. This may be described in a variety of ways, but the common denominator is that people feel as if they are floating away, leaving their body, becoming suddenly detached. The sensation is both weird and different; it is usually frightening. The person knows that something is definitely not right. Since these symptoms often accompany a fast or irregular pulse, the person may also be aware of a different or rapid heartbeat. This may be interpreted as a pounding in the chest, a fluttering feeling in the chest, or a sense of turning over inside. If the patient knows how to check his pulse, at that moment it will be abnormally fast or weak.

These symptoms may accompany the usual pain or discomfort that occurs in a heart attack or they may be the only symptoms which the person experiences. About ten percent of heart attacks are called "silent coronaries" because they are not associated with any form of pain. A patient of this type described these symptoms to me yesterday. He was at work at the time, sitting at his desk going over some papers.

He had the floating feeling and thought he might faint, but didn't. He left his job and drove himself to a hospital, where an electrocardiogram revealed that he was having a heart attack. When I asked him why he sought help, his interesting answer was that he knew something bad was happening to him and was afraid he was having a heart attack, even though he had no chest pain!

Shortness of Breath. A feeling of suffocation or shortness of breath may accompany a heart attack or occur in other heart conditions (primarily heart failure). If this symptom occurs along with the other symptoms that we have described, act as directed and get immediate medical help.

If shortness of breath occurs by itself, when is this significant? We'll proceed from the simple to the more complicated forms of this symptom. Most people from time to time sigh or take a deep breath. This is normal. Shortness of breath that occurs in an active person who is sitting down reading or eating is usually not significant. If he were to develop important shortness of breath, it would be much more likely to happen when he was working hard or walking rather than later on while he was resting. People with emphysema are often short of breath. This has usually developed over a long period of time and may have been associated with cigarette smoking and chronic coughing. Unless the shortness of breath suddenly increases, it is usually not an emergency.

Shortness of breath that occurs on mild exertion, such as walking half a block, climbing a flight of stairs, or carrying an object, may indicate heart trouble. This is particularly true if the subject was able to perform these same activities a short time beforehand without experiencing the symptom.

Any otherwise healthy person who mysteriously begins to develop this type of shortness of breath should consult his doctor. Any person who is known to have had any type of heart disease should notify his doctor of the problem today, not tomorrow.

Whenever any person awakens from sleep feeling short of breath, there is a good chance that he has trouble. I'm not referring to awakening from a dream and feeling frightened for a moment. I'm referring to waking up short of breath and either sitting up or propping up your head in order to breathe better. If you are really fighting for air and feel as though you have to get out of bed to walk or to get fresh air, this is very suggestive of heart failure, and you need help. With this set of circumstances, do awaken your doctor from his sleep, and don't wait until morning. A delay may result in things going from bad to worse. No doctor worth his salt values sleep more than the possibility of saving your life.

Rapid Heartbeat. If this symptom occurs with chest pain or pressure, indigestion, fainting, or shortness of breath, seek help immediately. You have a problem that requires attention—now.

A rapid heartbeat that occurs after strenuous exercise and quiets down to normal in a few minutes is not of concern. If you feel however that your heart is beating harder and longer than it used to with a familiar form of exertion, then although this is not an emergency situation, your heart deserves an examination. If on the other hand, your heart starts to beat hard and rapidly for no apparent reason, then you may have some form of tachycardia. Young people can often tolerate a tachycardia for up to several hours without otherwise feeling bad or getting into trouble. With persons middle-aged and older, the situation is going to depend on how strong oi how weak the heart is, and that may be impossible for the patient himself to judge.

A heart rate of 110 or 120 beats per minute may easily occur if a person is nervous, angry, excited, or feverish. This will rarely cause problems, unless it persists for days. Few middle-aged adults are going to be able to tolerate a heart rate of 140 to 150 or more for very long (minutes or hours) before they develop other symptoms of trouble. The first additional symptom that occurs could be weakness, chest pain, or shortness of breath.

The safest course to follow with any rapid heartbeat is to see your doctor. If it occurs for only brief periods of time (less than five minutes) and is not associated with other symptoms, the problem can wait until morning. If it persists for longer than five minutes, it is best to start moving toward help. Even though you may not develop other symptoms with a persisting tachycardia, it is highly desirable that a physician see you during an attack so that he can record an electrocardiogram to determine exactly what is happening and what should be done today and in the future to stop further attacks.

Sudden Weakness of an Arm or Leg, Sudden Loss of Eyesight or Speech. These are symptoms that occur when a person is suffering a stroke (damage to the brain due to blockage of an artery). Many strokes begin with a very temporary paralysis which completely disappears. The symptoms return in most cases to last longer and frequently result in permanent paralysis. Strokes can often be prevented, even at the stage of intermittent early symptoms, so don't delay— seek help.

It is difficult to understand why people often ignore the

early warning signs of a stroke, especially since modern medicine can often step in and prevent the final severe episode. The reason for this delay is probably a combination of ignorance and wishful thinking. Let's dispel both of these. If you suddenly develop weakness of a hand, arm, or leg, if you are suddenly dropping things from your hand or have trouble standing or walking, these may be warnings of a stroke that is destined to occur tonight or tomorrow unless you get help. The same thing applies to a temporary loss of speech, equilibrium, or eyesight (in one or both eyes, or a part of one eye). These symptoms represent a drastic change from normal. Something has to be wrong. Find out immediately, not tomorrow.

This information cannot be used as a substitute for seeing your own doctor and seeking his advice for problems. The main purpose of this information is to help the reader to realize that symptoms which are often cast aside as being unimportant are really very important.

20

Previews of Tomorrow

Medical knowledge has mushroomed over the past two decades, and we have many wonderful things to show for it. With the arrival of our new knowledge, we have also discovered great gaps in our information. The field of medical research has many more mysteries to unravel for us. In this chapter, we will view some of this research and some recent advances that have developed.

Our knowledge of risk factors in coronary heart disease needs strengthening. Although a great deal of supporting evidence has been gathered to justify proceeding with changes in our diet, smoking, and living habits, some people are withholding their support of these programs until further evidence is in. This is proper, as it forces us to continue research until not a shadow of a doubt exists as to the truth of these concepts.

In the meantime, however, we should not withhold this information from the public but should offer them the chance to make changes today that may influence their health tomorrow. An example of this lag of medical information occurred with Edward Jenner. He discovered that a vaccination with cowpox protected humans from contracting smallpox. The discovery occurred years before we knew the cause of smallpox or why the vaccination was effective, but fortunately, the use of the vaccination did not wait upon scientific answers as to "why and how."

The American Heart Association and the National Insti tutes of Health are proposing long-range studies of large groups of people to further clarify the risk factors. These studies will be valuable, and they may point up other un known factors that are significant.

An example of the type of research which is needed to further our understanding of basic types of heart disease follows. Drs. Swaye, Gifford, and Berrettoni of the Cleveland Clinic Foundation recently investigated effects of the salt in our diet on high blood pressure. One might have said that the study was unnecessary because everyone knows that eating too much salt will cause hypertension. The result of their program, which included the examination of 717 patients with hypertension and 819 people with normal blood pressures, was that there was no cause and effect relationship between using excess salt (defined in this study as adding salt to food before it was tasted) and subsequently developing hypertension. If a person already had high blood pressure, however, this habit often made the disease more severe and harder to control.

The search for an effective means of removing the deposits of atherosclerosis inside arteries continues. We are in desperate need of a medical "Drano®" so to speak. Various forms of surgery can remove localized obstructions in the larger blood vessels, but a chemical approach which would treat 100 percent of the obstructions, rather than the one percent now affected by surgery, is needed.

Dr. L. M. Morrison, director of the Institute for Arteriosclerosis Research at the Loma Linda University School of Medicine in California, reports in the December 1972 issue of *Cardiovascular and Metabolic Diseases* on his efforts along these lines. He has been working with a substance called chondroitin sulfate A (CSA) which he derives from the tracheal cartilage of the cow. Dr. Morrison treated 120 patients with coronary heart disease over a five-year period. One half the patients received daily doses of chondroitin sulfate A, and the other sixty patients did not. In all other respects, the two groups received similar treatment. At the end of the five years, the CSA group had had six cardiac incidents, while the control group had had thirty-nine. An acute cardiac incident was a heart attack, coronary insufficiency, or a threatened heart attack. In the CSA group there were only four deaths from coronary heart disease, and this compared to thirteen deaths in the control group. Dr. Morrison was unable to detect any side effects of the drug.

Chondroitin sulfate is a naturally occurring acid mucopolysaccharide found in all living creatures. The material is a basic ingredient of connective tissue, which is found throughout the body and binds other forms of tissue together. Dr. Morrison believes that a natural reserve of CSA in connective tissue becomes depleted with time, with the development of atherosclerosis in the arteries as one result. The CSA taken by the patients is believed to be capable of clearing away the atherosclerotic deposits in arteries.

A great deal of additional work will be necessary to clarify these findings, to substantiate them, and to determine the safety of the chemical. It is possible that CSA, or something like it, is on the horizon as a combined preventative and therapeutic measure to help in the battle against coronary heart disease and other forms of atherosclerosis.

When Coronary Care Units were established in hospitals throughout the United States, it was thought that the major step had been taken to decrease deaths from heart attacks. Although the statistics have been encouraging, we have recently found out that at least 50 percent of all deaths due to heart disease occur outside of hospitals. A report from Scotland on this subject set a record figure of 73 percent. Whichever figure is correct, the number is astronomical.

The next move to counteract this death rate was an attempt to move the hospital closer to the heart attack patient. Many large cities throughout the country, Los Angeles, Houston, Miami, and others, have established emergency medical rescue units. These rescue units are often built around the existing fire departments and consist of a special vehicle equipped with medical devices and manned by specially trained personnel. The public is told to call a central phone number in the case of a medical emergency. The rescue unit responds instead of a regular ambulance. If it is required when the unit reaches the scene, the personnel have been trained to give emergency treatment. Often an electrocardiogram can be taken on the spot and relayed by radio to a doctor standing by in a neighboring hospital. The doctor is in radio contact with the paramedical personnel and can give instructions. Many of the units carry defibrillators and emergency drugs for use as doctors' instructions indicate. A further refinement has occurred in Miami Beach, where physicians themselves ride in the vehicles.

Concern for early care has resulted in the establishment of emergency clinics in large stadiums, assuming that where large numbers of people congregate, heart attacks and sudden death will be more prone to occur. The Atlanta Stadium emergency service operates as follows: in the event a spectator collapses, a stadium area supervisor contacts the clinic by walkie-talkie. Aisle attendants start emergency cardiopulmonary resuscitation. A golf cart is dispatched to transport the stricken person to the clinic. In the clinic itself, further emergency equipment and personnel are available. An ambulance is on stand-by outside of the clinic to transport the patient to a nearby hospital.

Are these efforts paying off? What about the cost? As a rule of thumb, most larger cities have found that a comprehensive rescue squad costs the taxpayer one dollar per year for each of the community's inhabitants, so that a city of one million persons will spend about one million dollars a year for the service. A report covering five years of experience at the Atlanta Stadium, during which time there was a total attendance of nine million persons, revealed that thirteen spectators had had an apparent, sudden heart death. Three of these persons were successfully resuscitated. One of these resuscitations occurred prior to the establishment of the emergency service in 1970. During 1970 there were five apparent sudden deaths with two successful resuscitations. Results with the mobile rescue teams in various cities have been better, with many areas reporting over a 50 percent survival. Statistics will vary, depending on whether the survival rate is determined among all patients seen or only among those alive at the time the emergency team appears on the spot.

In Portland, Oregon emergency cardiac ambulance services have been provided without expense to the taxpayers. The local medical community helped to give special training to certain employees of the privately owned ambulance service in the city. Medical equipment including cardiac monitors and defibrillators were obtained from a private foundation.

A radio communication network had already been established between the ambulances and the local hospital. The service operates as follows: a special ambulance is dispatched for suspected heart cases. On arrival at the scene, the attendants check the patient's blood pressure, pulse, and electrocardiogram. If the patient is fibrillating, they can electrically defibrillate him on the spot and start cardiopulmonary resuscitation as needed. Recent approval has been obtained from the Oregon Board of Medical Examiners to allow these attendants to administer special cardiac drugs after checking the situation with a hospital-based doctor over the radio. The Portland program has been carried out without adding significantly to the fee ordinarily charged by the ambulance company for their calls.

Another variation has been developed at the Pennsylvania Hospital in Philadelphia. In this case the Mobile Coronary Care Unit is based at the hospital. When a call comes in, personnel from the hospital Coronary Care Unit are dispatched with the van. The obvious advantage of this system is that no special personnel are required, other than a driver. In addition, the same people who will be handling the patient inside the hospital are able to start their care at the patient's home or place of business, rather than an hour or so later, after transport and admission through an emergency room.

The Mobile Coronary Care Unit and Emergency Heart Rescue Units are a step in the right direction, but statistics tell us that between 40 and 50 percent of the patients who will die of a heart attack before they reach a hospital will do so within fifteen minutes from the onset of their symptoms. This means that patients must be made aware of the symptoms that indicate they need immediate help. The sooner the heart attack patient calls for assistance, the better his chances of survival will be.

This situation also points out the fact that still further steps will be necessary before we can significantly decrease the mortality associated with heart attacks. Medical researchers must discover ways to identify those who have a high risk of developing a heart attack and to pinpoint those who are particularly susceptible to fibrillation or cardiac standstill (the actual events which cause sudden death during the early phases of a heart attack). One possible solution might be for either the patient or a member of the family to immediately inject a drug which would decrease the chances of an erratic heartbeat. The ideal drug for this purpose has not been discovered yet.

Dr. M. Mirowski of Baltimore and others are at work on the development of a small, battery-powered, automatic defibrillator for temporary or permanent use in patients who have either had an episode or are at high risk of having ventricular fibrillation. This device will be similar in appearance and in method of attachment to a pacemaker. A catheter (wire) will run into the chamber of the right ventricle (one of the two main pumping units of the heart). The catheter will exit through a hole in a vein in the neck or shoulder. The actual defibrillating unit can be implanted under the skin on the front of the chest. If the patient develops ventricular fibrillation or another rapid heart rhythm which results in poor pumping of blood, the unit will sense this event and discharge a shock into the interior of the right ventricle. The energy required for this is tiny compared to the current necessary if the shock is applied to the outside of the chest. The unit will be able to recharge itself and deliver a second or third shock in seconds if needed. Further refinements in this unit might also incorporate the functions of a pacemaker. In this type of device, a differentiation could be made between too rapid a heartbeat (fibrillation or a fast tachycardia) and too slow a heartbeat (heart block or cardiac arrest). In the former circumstance, the unit would act as a defibrillator, in the latter event, as a pacemaker.

Turning our attention to investigations of another sort, let's look at the work that Dr. Wilbert Aronow and his group reported in the November 1972 issue of the *Annals of Internal Medicine*. They studied the effect of the air breathed by some heart patients, very special air—the air found around the Los Angeles freeway! Ten patients with angina pectoris were analyzed after spending 90 minutes driving around the freeway in heavy morning traffic with the car windows rolled down. They were later restudied after taking the same trip, but this time breathing compressed, purified air. The results of the first examination showed that the carbon monoxide level in their blood had risen strikingly and that they were able to perform far less activity than they had been able to before developing angina. Electrocardio-grams taken during the ride breathing outside air revealed significant changes that indicated a lack of oxygen nourish-ing the heart in three of the patients. The abnormal results were not encountered when the patients were breathing the purified, compressed air. The results were attributed directly to the carbon monoxide content of the freeway air. The source of the carbon monoxide was undoubtedly exhaust fumes from the automobiles.

Carbon monoxide combines with blood in such a way that the blood is able to carry less oxygen than it ordinarily would. This is the mechanism responsible for the develop-ment of angina with less than normal exertion. It is interesting that in seven of the ten patients, the blood levels of carbon monoxide were still significantly elevated two hours after they had left the freeway. It is apparent that physicians and patients will now have to consider the quality of air to which the patient is exposed when considering the various factors that may be aggravating his heart problem.

Unlimited horizons lie in the field of cardiac research. We will all reap the benefits of work being done in the areas of epidemiology, the effects of diet and hypertension on our hearts, and the development of new drugs and mechanical devices.

You can assist in the fight against heart disease by your vocal and financial support of those private agencies and government programs which are leading the way in research and public education. The American Heart Association, which has chapters in all states, is the leading example of private endeavor in heart research and education. Their programs are a great help in the continuing education of physicians and in the battle to get basic knowledge across to the public.

Glossary

aneurysm A sac formed by the dilatation of the walls of an artery, a vein, or a chamber of the heart. The sac is filled with blood and communicates freely with the general blood circulation.

angina pectoris A term that describes pain due to inadequate blood supply to the heart. The pain is usually in the chest or the arms and is frequently described as a squeezing, or pressure. It is usually only of several minutes duration and is relieved by rest or nitroglycerine.

aorta The large artery that carries blood away from the heart to the rest of the body. It arises from the left ventricle of the heart, runs through the chest and down the abdomen, giving off branches at various intervals. The vessel terminates when it divides into two branches that run down the legs.

arteriogram An x-ray of an artery. A dye that is vividly seen on x-ray film is injected into the artery and then one or more pictures are taken.

arteriosclerosis A group of disease processes that result in the narrowing of the lumen (passageway) of arteries. The blood vessels also become thickened and less elastic. Less than normal amounts of blood are able to flow through.

artery A blood vessel that carries blood from the heart to various parts of the body.

artificial heart-lung machine A device connected to a patient which temporarily replaces his heart. It pumps blood, removes carbon dioxide from the blood, and adds oxygen to it.

artificial pacemaker An electronic device that stimulates the heart with small electrical impulses to start each heartbeat.

atherosclerosis A type of arteriosclerosis. See arteriosclerosis.

atherosclerotic heart disease That type of heart disease caused by atherosclerosis. The end result of this disease may be a myocardial infarct (heart attack), heart failure, abnormal heart rhythms, or sudden death.

atherosclerotic plaque An individual patch of atherosclerosis. Also referred to as plaque.

atrial fibrillation A chaotic, irregular beating of the atria, resulting in an irregular and accelerated heartbeat. It is a common type of heartbeat that can be controlled by drugs.

atrial flutter A rapid and regular beating of the atria, resulting in an acceleration of the heartbeat.

atrium One of the two upper chambers of the heart. The right atrium receives blood from the body and delivers it to the right ventricle. The left atrium receives blood from the lungs and delivers it to the left ventricle.

auricle An appendage of each atrium. A small side pocket resembling the ear of a dog.

bundle branches (right and left) A segment of the heart's conduction system. Specialized portions of heart muscle that carry impulses through the ventricles to start each heartbeat.

bundle branch block An interruption in a particular portion of the system that transmits impulses through the heart. Similar to a broken wire.

cardiac reserve The reserve capacity of the heart to pump blood.

cardio-pulmonary resuscitation (CPR) A system of artificial respiration and circulation of the blood performed by persons or machines to maintain life in a patient whose heart has stopped beating or who has ceased breathing.

cholesterol A type of fat that is found in all animals as a normal part of the body. In the disease of atherosclerosis abnormal amounts of cholesterol accumulate in blood vessels.

complete heart block Complete interruption of the circuits that carry impulses from the atria to the ventricles. The result is a slowing of the heartbeat or cardiac arrest (absence of effective heartbeat).

conduction system Special portions of heart muscle carrying impulses through the heart that trigger heartbeats.

congenital heart disease Heart disease due to abnormal construction of the heart that has existed since birth.

coronary Frequently used as an informal term to mean a coronary occlusion or coronary thrombosis. See myocardial infarct.

coronary arteries The arteries that supply blood to the heart muscle. Two coronary arteries arise from the aorta immediately above the heart. The arteries encircle the heart and divide into many branches.

coronary arteriography An x-ray technique to obtain pictures of the coronary arteries.

coronary occlusion Obstruction or blockage of a coronary artery. This may result in a myocardial infarct. See myocardial infarct.

coronary thrombosis Obstruction of a coronary artery by a blood clot. This may result in a myocardial infarct. See myocardial infarct.

defibrillate To stop the process of fibrillation (abnormal heart beat). This may be accomplished with certain drugs or with an electrical shock applied over the chest of the patient by a special electronic apparatus.

diaphragmatic hernia An enlargement of the naturally occurring hole in the diaphragm (the sheet of muscle that separates the heart and lungs from the abdominal contents) through which the esophagus passes. The esophagus immediately empties into the stomach after it passes through the diaphragm. Because of the enlarged hole, a part of the stomach may slip up into the chest and produce pain.

edema An abnormal collection of fluid in the tissues of the body. This fluid usually obeys the laws of gravity and collects in the feet and ankles during the day when the patient is up and about.

electrocardiogram (ECG *or* EKG) A recording of the electrical events that occur in the heart during each heartbeat. Analysis of the recording can give information regarding the type of heartbeat, the speed of the beat, injury to the heart, enlargement of the heart, and the presence of a new or old myocardial infarct.

electrocardiograph An electronic apparatus that produces an electrocardiogram.

embolus Usually a blood clot that is carried by the circulation from one point to another and is finally forced into a small blood vessel in some part of the body. The embolus may completely block the vessel that it finally lodges in. Besides blood clots, other materials may become emboli, such as particles of fat, parasites, patches of atherosclerosis or even a bubble of air.

extrasystole A heartbeat occurring earlier than expected. Also called premature heartbeat.

fibrillation An irregular and disorganized heartbeat. See atrial fibrillation and ventricular fibrillation.

fluoroscope A screen that produces images of the internal structure of objects such as the human body that can be continuously examined with x-rays. To obtain a permanent record of the images, x-ray plates are used.

gangrene Death of body tissue due to inadequate blood flow to the tissue.

heart attack See myocardial infarct.

heart failure An inability of the heart to pump adequate amounts of blood. This may result in pulmonary edema, edema, or shock.

heart valve The heart has four valves, which open and close to insure that blood flows in and out only in the proper direction.

hiatal hernia See diaphragmatic hernia.

hypertension High blood pressure. Incorrectly used by some people to mean a state of anxiety or nervousness.

myocardial infarct (or *acute myocardial infarct*) The death of a portion of heart muscle due to an interruption in the blood supply. Coronary thrombosis and coronary occlusion are terms often used to signify this condition, although they actually only describe the obstruction of a coronary artery. This artery obstruction may or may not be followed by death of heart tissue, depending on the presence and adequacy of accessory or collateral arteries. The term heart attack is also used to describe a myocardial infarct.

pacemaker An impulse system of the heart that has the ability to initiate a heartbeat.

phlebitis See thrombophlebitis.

prothrombin time A test performed on a blood specimen that measures a blood clotting factor. The test is used to gauge the amount of certain drugs that are necessary to delay the clotting process in the body.

pulmonary edema The collection of fluid in the air spaces of the lungs. This is usually due to heart failure, but irritating gases such as chlorine can produce the same result. The patient experiences breathlessness as a result of this fluid.

pulmonary embolism Obstruction by an embolus of a large or small artery that carries blood through the lungs.

pulmonary infarct Death of a segment of lung tissue due to a pulmonary embolism. All pulmonary emoblisms do not produce pulmonary infarcts.

septal defects A hole in the partition that separates either the right atrium from the left or the right ventricle from the left. A ventricular septal defect may occur as the result of a myocardial infarct.

shock A state of pronounced depression of bodily processes associated with inadequate circulation of blood through the body. This is detected by a low or absent blood pressure. One cause of shock is defective pumping of blood by the heart. It is distinguished here from emotional shock, insulin shock, and therapeutic electrical shock.

sino-atrial node (or *sino-auricular node*) The primary natural pacemaker of the heart that usually initiates each heartbeat. It is located in the right atrium.

stroke Brain damage that is usually due to death of a piece of the brain because of an interruption in blood supply. It results in abnormal function of some part of the body, such as paralysis.

tachycardia Rapid heartbeat.

thrombophlebitis An inflammation of a vein that is usually accompanied by the formation of a blood clot in the vein.

thrombosis A blood clot.

vein A blood vessel that carries blood toward the heart from some part of the body.

ventricular aneurysm A saccular bulging of the heart wall that usually occurs as a result of a myocardial infarct.

ventricle Either of the two lower chambers of the heart, its main pumping chambers. The right ventricle pumps blood to the lungs, and the left ventricle pumps blood that has passed through the lungs to the rest of the body.

ventricular fibrillation An abnormal heart rhythm characterized by a quivering of the ventricles instead of a rhythmic contraction. The heart does not pump blood when the ventricles fibrillate, and death will occur within four or five minutes if it persists.

Index

Robert A. Miller, M.D.

Dr. Miller graduated from public schools in Key West, Florida, and in 1952 received an A.B. degree from Duke University. In 1956 he received his medical degree from George Washington University Medical School, Washington, D.C., at the age of 24.

Following a year of internship, he was commissioned as Captain in the Army Medical Corps. In his second year in the Army, Dr. Miller was a first-year medical resident in Tripler Army Hospital, Honolulu, and in the third and last year he was Medical Officer in that hospital.

For one year, 1961–1962, Dr. Miller was Chief Medical Resident at Jackson Memorial Hospital, Miami, Florida, and since 1962 he has been in private practice of Internal Medicine and Cardiology at the Naples Medical Center, Naples, Florida.

In 1967 he was Chief of Staff at Naples Community Hospital. He organized a Coronary Care Unit at that hospital in 1965 and has continued as Director of the Unit.